Substance Abuse

A Multi-Dimensional Assessment and Treatment Approach

Substance Abuse

A Multi-Dimensional Assessment and Treatment Approach

Penelope A. Moyers, EdD, OTR
Assistant Professor
University of Indianapolis
Indianapolis, Indiana

SLACK Incorporated, 6900 Grove Road, Thorofare, NJ 08086-9447

SLACK International Book Distributors

Japan
  Igaku-Shoin, Ltd.
  Tokyo International P.O. Box 5063
  1-28-36 Hongo, Bunkyo-Ku
  Tokyo 113
  Japan

Australia
  McGraw-Hill Book Company
  4 Barcoo Street
  Roseville East 2069
  New South Wales
  Australia

Canada
  McGraw-Hill Ryerson Limited
  300 Water Street
  Whitby, Ontario
  L1N 9B6

United Kingdom
  McGraw-Hill Book Company
  Shoppenhangers Road
  Maidenhead, Berkshire SL6 2QL
  England

In all other regions throughout the world, SLACK professional reference books are available through offices and affiliates of McGraw-Hill, Inc. For the name and address of the office serving your area, please correspond to

McGraw-Hill, Inc.
Medical Publishing Group
Attn: International Marketing Director
1221 Avenue of the Americas —28th Floor
New York, NY 10020
(212)-512-3955 (phone)
(212)-512-4717 (fax)

Editorial Director: Cheryl D. Willoughby
Publisher: Harry C. Benson

Cover design: Linda Baker, SLACK Inc.: reproduction of *The Way Out Discovered* by Paul Klée is with the permission of the estate of Paul Klée and the Artists' Rights Society, New York.

not my PF

Printed in the United States of America

Library of Congress Catalog Card Number: 88-43456

ISBN: 1-55642-084-6

Published by: SLACK Incorporated
               6900 Grove Road
               Thorofare, NJ 08086-9447

Last digit is print number: 10 9 8 7 6 5 4 3 2 1

CONTENTS

ACKNOWLEDGMENTS

Without the help of my husband David and my sons Patrick and Nathaniel, completion of this project would not have been possible. They offered me encouragement and enthusiasm as well as forgiveness when I spent long hours working. Cati Barrett, EdD, OTR, FAOTA designed many of the tables and figures in addition to making suggestions for structure and content. Zona Weeks, PhD, OTR, FAOTA and Trudy Martinez, MS, OTR provided assistance with organization. Shirley Bigna, MSLS, Assistant Director of the Krannert Memorial Library at the University of Indianapolis, indexed the book beautifully given the extremely short deadline. Sandy Clark helped me with some of the tables, but more importantly helped me with my schedule so that this book could be completed on time. Thank you for all the invaluable support.

INTRODUCTION

Newspaper headlines carry staggering figures on the number of drug-related deaths, injuries, automobile accidents, and health problems in the United States. Mothers Against Drunk Driving (MADD) wage their personal campaigns to "Stop the Maddness." Media personalities admonish the television public nightly to designate a driver, that drinking kills friendships, and to just say no. The war on drugs is a hot topic for politicians, religious leaders, teachers, and concerned citizens the world over as people become increasingly aware of this growing social crisis that threatens the fabric of society. What can occupational therapists do, with their focus on improving function, to treat substance abusers and to help such individuals return to responsible living?

This book has grown out of my years of experience in the field of mental health, particularly working with patients diagnosed with chemical dependency. Although my general knowledge of occupational therapy practice in mental health provided me with an excellent foundation for this work, I did at times feel ill prepared to address the unique needs of substance abusers. My colleagues who are specialists in the field of addiction have taught me a great deal. Interaction with patients demonstrated the shortcomings in my professional education with respect to the treatment of substance abuse, motivating me to learn from them all that I could. This book reflects my experience (both in private practice and in chemical dependency treatment programs), the insights I have gained in treating substance abusers, and my concerted efforts to study the field in depth.

The way in which occupational therapy benefits people suffering from substance abuse has yet to be studied beyond the superficial level. This book specifically addresses occupational therapy's role in the treatment of substance abusers. Occupational therapy frames of reference and methods appropriate for the treatment of substance abuse are examined as well. Succinctly, I am working from the assumption that these treatment approaches are applicable to persons who abuse a variety of substances.

To meet the objectives outlined, Chapter One, Substance Abuse and the Impact on Society, builds a foundation for the rest of the book by exploring the major concepts of substance abuse. It describes the prevalence and the effects of the problem upon society. Chapter Two, Differential Addiction States and Drugs of Choice, examines the relationship between typical coping styles and drug selection. It posits that substance abusers use drugs that augment the emotional state desired when experiencing stress. Stimulants are used by those individuals who prefer activation. Those who cope with stress by withdrawing into the self, typically abuse CNS depressants, such as alcohol, sedative-hypnotics, and opioids. Others avoid stress by abusing hallucinogens which compliment the desire to escape into fantasy.

Chapter Three, The Psychodynamics of Substance Abuse, explores the over-use of defense mechanisms by the substance abuser as a way to compensate for unmet dependency needs. These defense mechanisms, preferred by the substance abuser, require understanding by occupational therapists. Chapter Three also outlines three treatment levels that correspond to the changes in the substance abuser's reliance upon defense mechanisms that occur as the result of treatment.

Chapter Four, Clinical Reasoning and Substance Abuse, illustrates the process of choosing an appropriate psychosocial frame of reference that best addresses the critical issues of the substance abuser at each treatment level. This chapter describes matching the characteristics of the substance abuser with treatment variables to produce desired treatment outcomes. This discussion suggests evaluation tools that help the therapist determine the recovery stage and frames of reference appropriate for meeting the individual needs of the substance abuser.

Chapters Five through Seven analyze frames of reference and their applicability for treating problems inherent at each treatment level. They delineate specific treatment methodologies, corresponding to the principles of a particular frame of reference. Furthermore, they suggest various therapy groups according to the principles of each treatment level.

In Chapter Eight, Family Treatment and Occupational Therapy, the three treatment levels organize occupational therapy designed for family members of substance abusers. It delineates a treatment approach that closely corresponds to the treatment principles of the substance abuser. Chapter Nine, Sandra: A Case Example, integrates the concepts presented in previous chapters.

Finally, Chapter Ten, Trends in Substance Abuse Rehabilitation, examines current issues in the field of substance abuse and advocates directions for research. The goal is to promote functional performance as an excellent avenue for making an important contribution to the study of substance abuse and its treatment.

It is the desire of this author to stimulate more interest in the practice of occupational therapy in the area of substance abuse. Drug abuse certainly is a growing national health problem that affects all specializations in occupational therapy. For example, the treatment of a pediatric patient suffering from a handicapping condition is negatively affected by alcoholic parents. An intoxicated adolescent may suffer a head injury resulting from driving while abusing drugs. Even though no longer drinking, a chronic alcoholic suffering from a stroke may be unable to participate adequately in the stroke rehabilitation program due to interfering, alcoholic-like defensive behavior. A wife, hospitalized for depression, may have difficulty responding to treatment because of a lack of focus on the complications arising from her husband's cocaine addiction.

By the end of this book, the importance of examining the special needs of the substance abuser and the family as well as determining the best treatment approach that produces the desired outcomes should be clear. Occupational therapy's focus on functional performance enhances the substance abuser's return to optimal social functioning.

Substance Abuse and the
Impact on Society

INTRODUCTION

Substance abuse has a distinct influence on society that goes beyond the suffering of the individual. The family experiences consequences of living with a substance abuser that could possibly impact succeeding generations. The employed substance abuser negatively affects coworkers and potentially decreases the quality of products purchased by consumers. This, of course, is in addition to the cost of absenteeism and the health care expenditures related to the physical side-effects of long-term addiction. Society also spends exorbitant amounts for rehabilitation, law enforcement, and prevention of substance abuse. The effects of substance abuse upon society can be listed almost endlessly, but the point remains that the problem is broad in scope.

This chapter explores several aspects of substance abuse that underlie the importance of occupational therapists becoming more involved in this area of mental health practice. Background information is provided regarding prevalence of substance abuse in the United States. Basic concepts and terminology are briefly reviewed followed by a discussion of the controversy related to the definition of substance abuse. Next, the problems of comorbidity and dual diagnoses are examined.

Occupational therapy issues that could potentially affect involvement in the treatment of substance abuse are reviewed. Occupational therapy offers a functional perspective that is often ignored by other treatment professionals, but is important for the substance abuser's community adjustment as a sober member of society. This chapter concludes by examining the differential roles of disciplines involved in the treatment of substance abuse and the way in which occupational therapy compliments the functional perspectives of other disciplines.

◆ PREVALENCE AND FREQUENCY OF USE ◆

Statistics overwhelmingly substantiate the problem of alcoholism and abuse of chemicals in society. An Ecological Catchment Area Study found that substance abuse disorders were the second most common psychiatric diagnostic category.[1] For men aged 16 to 64, substance abuse disorders were the most prominent diagnosis. Among the substance abuse disorders, however, alcohol-related disorders were two to three times as prevalent. It is estimated that there are 13 million persons with alcoholism in the United States.[2]

According to a 1984 population survey of alcohol use, effects of age and sex distributions on drinking patterns, frequency of high intake occasions, and drinking problems were as expected.[3] For males, problematic drinking was highest for persons aged 18 to 29 years old. Men in their forties, though, seemed to be more vulnerable for experiencing tangible consequences of drinking. Examples of tangible consequences included job difficulties, marital discord, and legal problems.

Women, on the other hand, had rather constant proportions of problem drinkers across age groups. Women aged 18 to 29 seemed to be the most vulnerable in terms of suffering tangible consequences of drinking.[3] In general, drinking problems were more commonly reported by male drinkers than female drinkers and by younger drinkers than by older drinkers. Those who drank five or more drinks in a single day, as often as once per week, were the most likely to experience problematic drinking and tangible consequences.

According to *Medical World News*, between four million and five million people were regular users of cocaine during the early 1980s, with approximately one million estimated as being profoundly dependent upon the drug.[4] At that time, about 22 million people in the United States had tried cocaine at least once. The number of current users of cocaine has dropped significantly from 5.8 million in 1985 to 1.6 million in 1990.[5] The number of current cocaine users in 1991 was estimated as being approximately the same as the estimate for 1990. Even though current use of cocaine has declined over the last five years, however, frequent or more intense use of cocaine has not changed significantly. One million people used crack in 1991, the same number as in 1988 and 1990.

It seems that the downward trend in cocaine use has begun to level off, but related deaths and weekly use have not changed. Cocaine abusers are using the drug in large and dangerous quantities.[5] According to the Drug Abuse Warning Network, cocaine-related emergencies and deaths increased fivefold during the period between 1983 and 1988.[6] By 1989, cocaine-related emergency room visits fell by 27 percent (11,145 to 8,135), but the number of cocaine-related deaths increased (2,254 to 2,496).[7]

Data from the 1984, 1988 and 1991 Household Surveys on Drug Abuse showed a trend in decreased recreational use of heroin, marijuana, and phencyclidine, dropping from 14.9 percent in 1985 to 6.8 percent in 1991.[5,8] Marijuana is the most widely abused illegal drug in the United

States, with an estimated 67.7 million Americans having used the drug at least once in their lifetime.[5] Even though recreational use has decreased, however, there is an observed trend for increased drug use in the inner cities. This urban trend is characterized by substance abuse starting at a younger age, with addiction occurring earlier as well. Drug users include 15.4 percent of persons between the ages of 18 and 25; 16.8 percent of unemployed persons; 9.4 percent of blacks; and 8.1 percent of persons in large metropolitan areas in the West.[5]

◆ BASIC CONCEPTS ◆

Before proceeding further, it is useful to explore the definitions of substance abuse. The revised third edition of the *Diagnostic and Statistical Manual of Mental Disorders* (DSM-III-R) distinguishes between psychoactive substance abuse and dependence on the basis of presenting symptomatology.[9] Dependence involves a pattern of pathological and compulsive drug use manifested by intoxication. There is an inability to reduce and/or stop ingestion of the substance despite periodic attempts to control use or the presence of disturbing complications. [10] Severity of dependence is rated in terms of mild, moderate, severe, in partial remission or in full remission according to specific criteria.

Abuse is differentiated from dependence primarily by fewer symptoms shown in abuse and by the individual not ever having previously met the criteria for dependence. Abuse involves maladaptive use of substances rather than compulsive use, which is reflective of dependence. Additionally, abuse does not involve either the development of tolerance or withdrawal symptoms.

Other substance-related disorders involve either drug intoxication or drug withdrawal, leading to organic mental disorders (eg. alcohol withdrawal delirium, amphetamine intoxication, or cocaine delusional disorders). The particular substance used determines the characteristics of the withdrawal syndrome. The most frequent withdrawal symptoms include anxiety, restlessness, irritability, insomnia, and impaired attention.

◆ DIAGNOSTIC ISSUES ◆

The changes brought forth by the DSM-III-R diagnostic delineation of substance dependence reflect a movement toward "a multifocal approach and away from reliance solely on physiological dependence."[11] Diagnosis, in addition to the typical concern with the nature and severity of dependence, also considers the kinds and degrees of disability, and the personal and environmental factors influencing substance use. Substance dependence is no longer viewed as an all-or-nothing process, but one that exists in degrees. The concept that substance dependence as a syndrome is generic to all psychoactive substances improves comparisons among a variety of drugs along the same symptomatologic dimensions.[12]

Controversy exists, however, regarding the difficulty in making a diagnostic determination between abuse and dependence. The DSM-III-R definition of dependence is primarily "conceptualized as compulsive use, characterized by cognitive, behavioral, and physiological aspects."[13] Consequently, physiological dependence and tolerance are not the major diagnostic criteria. If at least three of the nine possible DSM-III-R criteria are met, it is possible for an individual to be diagnosed as substance dependent without ever exhibiting tolerance or withdrawal. Critics have expressed concern regarding the resulting increased heterogeneity of dependence and the reduced saliency of the abuse concept.

Schuckit, Sisook and Mortola explored the clinical significance of differentiating between alcohol abuse and dependence.[14] Male alcoholics diagnosed with abuse and those with dependence were virtually identical at admission and during the one-year follow-up. Early life antisocial problems were similar as were drug use patterns and psychiatric histories. The only significant difference was in the number of drinks per drinking day, but not in the number of drinking days.

Gold and Dackis reported that substance abuse is still a common cause of misdiagnosis.[15] Many studies substantiate that primary care physicians have not been successful at diagnosing and treating patients with substance abuse and dependence. [16-18] Genetic research may lead to alternative methods of defining diagnostic categories for substance abuse and dependence. Kleinman stated that specific biochemical abnormalities will eventually be discovered among addicts.[19] Instead of using symptoms, as in DSM-III-R criteria, diagnosis could be based on use and family history.

For example, there are at least two forms of alcoholism with a substantial genetic basis, ie. "male-limited" (genetically transmitted through the father) and "matrilineal" (genetically transmitted by the mother).[20-23] Recently, researchers have detected an allelic (ie. genes located in the same position on a pair of chromosomes), association with the dopamine D2 receptor gene with susceptibility to at least one form of alcoholism.[24] As described by Goodwin, this genetic form of alcoholism, often referred to as "primary alcoholism," has an early onset, severe symptomatology, and requires extensive, early treatment.[22] Primary alcoholism does not result from a concomitant psychiatric illness and is usually associated with males.[25]

Reich, Cloninger, Van Eerdewegh, Rice and Mullaney compared the frequency of alcoholism in first degree relatives and spouses of alcoholics with the age-specific lifetime population rates determined by the Epidemiological Catchment Area Study.[1, 26] The comparison illustrated that despite an increasing population prevalence of alcoholism in general, the familial aggregation of alcoholism was maintained. The majority of alcoholics were from alcoholic families.

The genetic component of substance abuse is multifactional and complex. The interaction between genetics and the environment impacts the frequency and amount of the drug consumed, the development of tolerance, and the type of medical complications suffered.[27] It is also strongly suspected that different risk factors lead to different forms of substance abuse. Persons with early onset should be studied apart from those with late onset. Likewise, those with antisocial personality should be examined separately from those without, men apart from women, and those with a family history distinctly from those with no family history.[28] Substance abuse definitely is not a unitary condition.

◆ COMORBIDITY ◆

There is a high comorbidity rate between substance abuse and other psychiatric diagnoses. The Epidemiological Catchment Area (ECA) study determined that 10 percent of the total sample had a diagnosis of alcoholism, which was the most prevalent diagnosis.[29] Almost half of those reporting symptoms of alcoholism (47 percent) had another psychiatric diagnosis. In fact, they were more likely than the sample with other psychiatric diagnoses to have dual diagnoses.

Most of this comorbidity for alcoholics was accounted for by drug abuse and antisocial personality disorder. Mania was also strongly associated with alcoholism, but depression and dysthymia were not.[29] This is in contrast to Weissman and Meyers' survey that indicated 55 percent of the alcoholics had a concurrent depressive diagnosis, and out of that percentage 60 percent suffered from a primary depression that preceded the onset of alcoholism.[30] Abuse of substances in general, including alcohol, has been associated with affective disorders, anxiety disorders, eating disorders, schizophrenia, phobic disorders, posttraumatic stress disorder, and organic brain syndromes.[31, 32] In adolescents, substance use is additionally associated with conduct disorder and attention deficit disorder.[33]

The National Institute of Mental Health declared the study of dual diagnoses a priority. Research indicates that 87 percent of 92,509 cases with a primary mental disorder also had a secondary diagnosis of alcohol dependence or nondependent alcohol abuse.[31] These dually diagnosed patients constitute 30 to 50 percent of psychiatric populations and up to 80 percent of substance abusers.[32] This prevalence raises concern, especially since substance abuse is often masked by the symptoms of the primary or secondary mental illness.

◆ OCCUPATIONAL THERAPY ◆

Due to the incidence of drug use in the United States, substance abuse deserves attention from occupational therapists. Regardless of the practice specialty area, substance abuse is likely to influence, at some point, the occupational therapist's professional experience. The occupational therapist may have a family member or may be working with treatment team members that are abusing substances. In the process of providing treatment for a patient's medical or psychological condition, the occupational therapist may inadvertently be struggling with complications arising from the patient's undiagnosed substance abuse. The patient's family may abuse substances and the resulting impaired family dynamics could interfere with treatment progress in occupational therapy. The negative effects of substance abuse upon society as a whole are extensive and require recognition from occupational therapists in terms of conducting research and designing effective treatment strategies.

The diagnostic criteria for substance abuse is in a continuing state of evolution. Unfortunately, substance abuse is still being defined in terms of quantitative amounts of the particular drug consumed in a given time period. This definition is being questioned due to the considerable variability in patterns of use across individuals. Diagnosis remains unclear due to the lack of definitive understanding regarding the biological and behavioral aspects of substance abuse related disorders.

Health professionals generally understand that diagnosis should be specific, comprehensive and based on etiology. When this is true, diagnosis implies a treatment approach. The lack of a truly comprehensive model for explaining substance abuse seriously hampers diagnostic and treatment efforts. For example, because familial alcoholism appears to have a strong genetic component, abstinence is probably the best possible treatment goal.[34] Some substance abusers may have neuropsychological impairments requiring remediation of cognitive deficits. Other substance abusers, due to psychostructural deficits (ego weakness or antisocial personality), could possibly benefit from a psychodynamic approach.

Occupational therapy and other rehabilitation services bring a functional perspective to the treatment of substance abuse that is not dependent upon the medical diagnosis. This functional orientation is often lacking when rehabilitation professionals are excluded from the treatment program. Einstein, Wolfson and Gecht completed a study of alcoholism treatment personnel and found that these personnel tended to focus on only one aspect of the alcoholism syndrome, ie. the problems related to personal maladjustment.[35] These researchers and others do not feel it is reasonable to expect that effective treatment and/or prevention of a complex condition like alcoholism could occur with simplistic approaches.[35,36] A singular focus fails to address such problems as legal, social and vocational difficulties.[36]

The occupational therapy functional assessment provides information regarding the substance abuser's strengths and weaknesses in performing tasks inherent in culturally relevant roles.[37] An occupational therapy diagnosis is formulated that accurately reflects the dysfunctional and functional abilities of the substance abuser. The occupational therapy diagnosis describes the occupational component dysfunction/function, which involves the underlying factors of sensorimotor, cognitive, or psychosocial aspects of functioning. The diagnosis also indicates the occupational performance dysfunction/function or those specific activities of daily living (ADL), work or leisure tasks important to the substance abuser's community adjustment. Ultimately, the occupational therapy diagnosis describes the occupational role dysfunction/function or the substance abuser's intact or impaired work, leisure, family and community roles.

More specifically, the occupational therapist determines the way in which the pathology associated with substance abuse impacts the cognitive, sensory processing, motor, emotional and social functioning of the individual. The occupational therapy diagnosis does not stop at this point, but includes the way in which these components of functioning influence the individual's ability to complete routine daily tasks associated with the person's roles in the community.[37] For instance, a substance abuser who has problems with memory may forget some of the tasks assigned by the supervisor in a work setting. The substance abuser might also leave out essential steps required for the proper completion of each job task. Because of these problems experienced on the job, the work role of the substance abuser may be impaired, creating problems for future independence in community living.

The occupational therapy diagnosis directs treatment planning by targeting behaviors for change. Change comes about by designing treatment consistent with theoretical principles described by a particular psychosocial frame of reference. A frame of reference delineates therapeutic action specific to an individual practitioner's domain of concern or area of expertise.[38] Because the frame of reference guides selection of treatment approaches consistent with selected theories, a linking of theory and clinical practice occurs. According to Mosey, the structure of a frame of reference involves the following: a) the theory base, b) function/dysfunction continuums, c) behavioral indications of function and dysfunction, and d) postulates regarding change.[39]

In this book, several frames of reference are described in terms of the importance for guiding the treatment of substance abusers throughout several stages of recovery. These frames of reference include: a) management of cognitive disabilities, b) action-consequence (behavioral), c) cognitive-behavioral, d) model of human occupation, and e) object relations (psychoanalytical).

Occupational therapy addresses the functional problems influenced by substance abuse. Emphasis is placed upon community adjustment to a drug free life. This adjustment or adaptation depends upon the individual's ability to sustain appropriate activity levels, access social networks, develop intimate relationships, achieve economic sufficiency and control abstinence.[40] The functional abilities of the substance abuser ultimately determine the quality of community adjustment to sobriety. Occupational therapy intervention involves augmenting existing functional skills, modifying inappropriate behaviors, and teaching new functional skills that are considered relevant in a variety of settings by the substance abuser. Occupational therapy also facilitates the substance abuser's motivation for change.[40] The home environment is analyzed for support of the substance abuser's improved functional behavior.

◆ MULTIDISCIPLINARY TREATMENT TEAM ◆

Adaptive functioning is an important factor in determining length of psychiatric hospitalization.[41] According to Fine, "This focus on function emphasizes the strong role that occupational therapy should play in program development in mental health settings."[42] Because functioning is a complicated and broad area of concern, treatment by one discipline is rarely effective. Assessing functional problems and intervening in order to improve performance in cultural roles, depends upon the multiple perspectives of a multidisciplinary treatment team, the substance abuser who is the object of treatment, and the family and other significant members of the social system. As Dickie and Robertson point out, "The specialization of each discipline and the unique understanding of each individual can offer in-depth pictures of different aspects of functioning, such as physical capacities, daily living skills, performance in the environmental context, fulfillment of cultural expectations, and social interaction."[43]

Disciplines included in the multidisciplinary treatment team depend upon a number of external and internal factors specific for each substance abuse treatment program. External factors include political, economic and demographic issues. The internal factors of a treatment program include the size of the facility, the nature of the services provided (detoxification, inpatient or outpatient), the philosophy of the setting, and available resources (grants, third-party insurance coverage or governmental financial support).

In addition to occupational therapy, typical disciplines involved in the treatment of substance abuse include psychiatrists, nurses, psychologists, social workers, chaplains and a number of activity therapy personnel. Lay persons or recovering substance abusers usually play a strong role in most substance abuse treatment programs.

The psychiatrist assesses and treats the individual's medical and psychological problems experienced during recovery. Often these professionals assume the coordinating functions for the treatment team by determining the necessary psychological, neurological or medical interventions. Psychologists are also concerned with the individual's neurological and psychological functioning. The nursing staff, in conjunction with physicians, monitor the medical status and treat the medical needs of the individual, especially those problems related to detoxification and the long-term physical side-effects related to chronic use of drugs.

The lay counselors focus on the 12-step issues of Alcoholics Anonymous (AA) for each individual through the use of educational groups. The substance abuser's loss of control over the chemical and the consequences that the addiction has had on the individual's life are also addressed within these groups. Facilitating involvement in self-help programs is also accomplished by supervising attendance at Narcotics Anonymous or Alcoholics Anonymous (NA/AA) meetings.

The social worker usually acts as the liaison between the family, the substance abuser and the treatment team. Social workers often implement the family education programs along with the family therapy sessions. Chaplains address the spiritual aspects of the recovery process. Activity therapy personnel, such as recreational therapists, are responsible for normalizing leisure functioning. The substance abuser is assisted in obtaining new alternatives to the previous drug-related lifestyle.

The multidisciplinary approach to treatment meshes many different components into a comprehensive and multifaceted intervention style.[44] Even though each member of the treatment team offers a different perspective, there is overlap among the roles of the various disciplines as well. Because each of the disciplines claims to facilitate improved functioning in the substance abuser, there may seem to be a duplication of services at first glance. Functioning, as described earlier, has complex meanings and therefore requires a multifaceted and overlapping approach.

By way of example, note that occupational therapy overlaps with psychology in addressing the psychological and neurological components of functioning. Similarly, nursing and occupational therapy may overlap by focusing on the tasks associated with activities of daily living (hygiene, dressing or feeding). Occupational therapy and recreational therapy may overlap by their common concerns for necessary changes in the leisure role required for independent community living.

Because of the overlap among the various disciplines on the substance abuse treatment team, confusion regarding professional boundaries may result. According to Rogers and Holmes, the concept of functioning in occupational therapy is unique in comparison with the functional definitions offered by other disciplines. In occupational therapy, the concept of functioning includes the simultaneous impact of component abilities and task performance upon community role functioning.[37]

For instance, even though nursing and occupational therapy both focus on activities of daily living, the occupational therapist analyzes how neurocognitive defects affect routine ADL performance. In this respect, the ADL task is simplified to accommodate the cognitive limitations of the addict. The substance abuser's role in self-care is modified in the community by arranging for ongoing supervision of ADL performance. The substance abuser's family members are taught how to redesign the home environment to provide the cognitive cues necessary for independent ADL task performance. Consequently, as Rogers and Holm have noted, "Recognition of the uniqueness of OT and how the OT domain of practice overlaps with the domains of other professions can help one be more articulate in explaining OT to others—patients, students, legislators, or third-party payers."[37]

◆ CONCLUSIONS ◆

The professional issues outlined in this chapter are addressed by this book, thereby demonstrating that occupational therapy is a necessary part of the treatment regimen for substance abuse. The role of occupational therapy is clarified and a theoretical approach for the treatment of substance abuse is delineated. This theoretical approach is rooted in developing theories of substance abuse as well as in occupational therapy theories of psychosocial dysfunction. Applications to a variety of treatment settings are explained, thereby enhancing the versatility of occupational therapy.

A functional treatment emphasis is advocated that promotes occupational therapy as a cost-effective service. Existing research is examined in order to determine valid treatment methodologies and to outline a specific research focus for the future. It is hoped that the information presented in this book will favorably enhance the quality of occupational therapy services provided to persons suffering from substance abuse.

References

1. Regier DA, Myers JK, Kramer M, Robins LN, Blazer DG, Hough RL, Eaton W, Locke BZ: The NIMH epidemiologic catchment area program. *Arch Gen Psychiatry* 41: 934-941, 1984.
2. Kaplan HI, Sadock BJ: *Synopsis of Psychiatry, Behavioral Sciences, Clinical Psychiatry,* 5th ed. Baltimore: Williams & Wilkins, 1988.
3. Hilton ME: Drinking patterns and drinking problems in 1984: Results from a general population survey. *Alcohol Clin Exp Res* 11(2): 167-175, 1987.
4. Cocaine is a killer, specialists warn, as drug supplies rise and prices drop. *Medical World News* (May 28): 16-18, 1984.
5. *National Household Survey on Drug Abuse.* Rockville, MD: National Institute of Mental Health, 1991.

6. Kozel NJ: Epidemiology of drug abuse in the United States: A summary of methods and findings. *Bulletin of the Pan American Health Organization* 24: 53-62, 1990.

7. Culhane C: Drug use falls but deaths are up. *US Journal,* Dec 11: 11, 1990.

8. Adams E: *Overview of selected drug trends.* Rockville, MD: National Institute on Drug Abuse, Publication RP0731, 1989.

9. American Psychiatric Association: *Diagnostic and Statistical Manual of Mental Disorders,* 3d ed. rev. Washington, DC: Author, 1987.

10. Smith D, Milkman H, Sunderwirth S: Addictive disease: Concept and controversy. In Milkman H and Shaffer H (Eds.): *The Addictions.* Lexington, MA: D.C. Heath and Company, 1985, pp. 145-159.

11. Kaufman E, McNaul JP: Recent developments in understanding and treating drug abuse and dependence. *Hosp Community Psychiatry* 43(3): 223-236, 1992, p. 227.

12. Babor TF, Orrok B, Liebiwitz N, et al: From basic concepts to clinical reality: Unresolved issues in the diagnosis of dependence. *Recent Dev Alcohol* 8: 85-104, 1990.

13. Schuckit M, Helzer J, Crowley T, Nathan P, Woody G, Dairs W: Substance use disorders. *Hosp Community Psychiatry* 42(5): 471-473, 1991, p. 471.

14. Schuckit MA, Zisook S, Mortola J: Clinical implications of DSM-III diagnoses of alcohol abuse and alcohol dependence. *Am J Psychiatry* 142(12): 1403-1408, 1985.

15. Gold MS, Dackis CA: Role of the laboratory in the evaluation of suspected drug abuse. *J Clin Psychiatry* 47: 17-23, 1986.

16. Moore RD, Malitz FE: Underdiagnosis of alcoholism by residents in an ambulatory medical practice. *J Med Educ* 61: 46-52, 1986.

17. Chappel JN, Schnoll S: Physician attitudes: Effect on the treatment of chemically dependent patients. *JAMA* 237: 2318-2319, 1977.

18. Ramsay A, Vredenburgh J, Gallagher RM: Recognition of alcoholism among patients with psychiatric problems in a family practice clinic. *J Fam Pract* 17: 829-832, 1983.

19. Kleinman P: Onset of addiction: A first attempt at prediction. *Int J Addict* 13: 1217-1235, 1978.

20. Cloninger R, Bohman M, Sigvaardson S: Inheritance of alcohol abuse: Cross-fostering analyses of adopted men. *Arch Gen Psychiatry* 38: 861-867, 1981.

21. Goodwin DW: *Is Alcoholism Hereditary?* New York: Oxford University Press, 1976.

22. Goodwin DW: Alcoholism and heredity. *Arch Gen Psychiatry* 36: 57-61, 1979.

23. Petrakis PL: *Alcoholism: An Inherited Disease.* Washington, DC: National Institute on Alcohol Abuse and Alcoholism, 1985.

24. Blum K, Noble EP, Sheridan PJ, Montgomery A, Ritchie T, Jagadeeswaran P, Nogami H, Briggs AH, Cohn JB: Allelic association of human dopamine D2 receptor gene in alcoholism. *JAMA* 263: 2055-2060, 1990.

25. Tarter R, Alterman A, Edwards K: Vulnerability to alcoholism in men: A behavior-genetic perspective. *J Stud Alcohol* 46: 259-261, 1985.

26. Reich T, Cloninger CR, Van-Eerdewegh P, Rice JP, Mullaney J: Secular trends in the familial transmission of alcoholism.*Alcohol Clin Exp Res* 12(4): 458-464, 1988.

27. Begleiter H, Porjesz B: Potential biological markers in individuals at high risk for developing alcoholism. *Alcohol Clin Exp Res* 12(4): 488-493, 1988.

28. Donovan JM: An etiologic model of alcoholism. *Am J Psychiatry* 143(1): 1-11, 1986.

29. Helzer JE, Pryzbeck TR: The co-occurrence of alcoholism with other psychiatric disorders in the general population and its impact on treatment. *J Stud Alcohol* 49(3): 219-224, 1988.

30. Weissman MM, Meyers JK: Clinical depression in alcoholism. *Am J Psychiatry* 137: 372-373, 1980.

31. Kiesler CA, Simpkins CG, Morton, TL: Prevalence of dual diagnoses of mental and substance abuse disorders in general hospitals. *Hosp Community Psychiatry* 42(4): 400-403, 1991.

32. Kosten TR, Kleber HD: Differential diagnosis of psychiatric comorbidity in substance abusers. *J Sub Abuse Treat* 5: 201-206, 1988.

33. Bukstein OG, Brent DA, Kaminer Y: Comorbidity of substance abuse and other psychiatric disorders in adolescents. *Am J Psychiatry* 146: 1131-1141, 1989.

34. Donovan JM: An etiologic model of alcoholism. *Am J Psychiatry* 143(1): 1-11, 1986.

35. Einstein S, Wolfson E, Gecht P: What matters in treatment: Relevant variables in alcoholism. *Int J Addict* 5: 54-67, 1970.

36. Pemper K: Dimensions of change in the improving alcoholic. *Int J Addict* 11: 641-649, 1976.

37. Rogers J, Holm MB: The therapist's thinking behind functional assessment I. In CB Royeen (Ed.): *AOTA Self Study Series Assessing Function.* Rockville, MD: American Occupational Therapy Association, 1989, pp. 1-32.

38. Denton PL, Skinner ST: Selecting a frame of reference/practice model. In SC Robertson (Ed.): *Mental Health FOCUS Skills for Assessment and Treatment*. Rockville, MD: American Occupational Therapy Association, 1988, pp. 100-108.

39. Mosey AC: *Occupational therapy: Configuration of a Profession*. New York: Raven Press, 1981.

40. Palmer F: *The Present Context of Service Delivery. In SC Robertson (Ed.): Mental Health FOCUS Skills for Assessment and Treatment*. Rockville, MD: American Occupational Therapy Association, 1988, pp. 28-36.

41. Mezzich JE, Coffman GA: Factors influencing length of hospital stay. *Hosp Community Psychiatry* 36(12): 1262-1270.

42. Fine SB: Trends in mental health. In SC Robertson (Ed.): *Mental Health SCOPE Strategies, Concepts, and Opportunities for Program Development and Evaluation in Occupational Therapy Curriculum*. Rockville, MD: American Occupational Therapy Association, 1986, pp. 19-32.

43. Dickie VA, Robertson SC: Occupational therapy update: Perspectives on human functioning. *Hosp Community Psychiatry* 42(6): 575-576, 1991, p. 576.

44. Klein JM, Miller SI: Three approaches to the treatment of drug addiction. *Hosp Community Psychiatry* 37(11): 1083-1085, 1986.

Differential Addiction States
and Drugs of Choice

INTRODUCTION

Occupational therapy for substance abusers is likely to be more effective when the therapist uses knowledge about the physiological actions of a variety of commonly abused substances in selecting the best treatment approach. This chapter analyzes the tendency for specific drugs to be abused in a manner that is consistent with the abuser's preferred coping style. The relationship between drug choice and coping style is important for understanding differential treatment needs. Therefore, the major drug classifications of alcohol, sedative-hypnotics, stimulants, opioids, and hallucinogens are examined. Although there are similarities that govern treatment for all substance abusers, incorporating specific approaches for the heroin addict, for example, versus those techniques used for the amphetamine abuser is important.

◆ METHODS OF DEALING WITH STRESS ◆

Addiction involves compulsion, loss of control, and continuation in spite of harmful consequences. Milkman and Sunderwirth define addiction as "self-induced changes in neurotransmission which result in problem behaviors."[1] This definition includes interrelated factors of personal responsibility (self-inducement), biochemical effects (neurotransmission) and social reactions (problem behaviors).

Self-inducement is reinforced over time as the substance abuser uses specific chemicals to produce the necessary neurotransmission consistent with the feeling desired. It is apparent through research that the type of drug used depends on the user.[1-3] In fact, Milkman and Frosch determined that there is a strong relationship between personality and the drug of choice.[4] They maintain that individuals prefer drugs that complement the level of arousal routinely utilized in coping with stress.[4] For example, individuals who prefer active involvement during times of stress may be prone to the pharmacological effects of stimulants. This is in contrast to individuals who cope by seeking relaxation. The withdrawing from stress is facilitated by use of satiation- or sedative-type drugs. Those who approach stress through escape into fantasy may choose hallucinogenic drugs.

The drug of choice changes the pattern of neurotransmission by either increasing or decreasing the rate of nerve impulse transmission. This change in rate is dependent upon the interaction of the drug at the synaptic junction. Cocaine tends to prevent the neurotransmitter (norepinephrine) from being reabsorbed into the presynaptic terminal. As a result, more norepinephrine, an excitatory neurotransmitter, is available for attachment to receptor sites. Rate of neurotransmission is thereby increased. This increased rate of neurotransmission produces an increase in the individual's state of arousal.[5, 6]

A slightly different process occurs when ingesting sedative type drugs. In this case, the individual seeks a substance that decreases the rate of neurotransmission. Opiates attach to receptor sites at the presynaptic terminal that decrease the release of the neurotransmitter.[7] Decreasing the release of neurotransmitters reduces the rate of neurotransmission. Slower neurotransmission decreases physiological arousal, which is the desired behavior.

The effects of hallucinogens upon neurotransmission are less well understood than the effects of opiates and stimulants. Hallucinogens facilitate escape into fantasy through some method of interfering with the normal mechanism of neurotransmission. In fact, there is a close relationship between the chemical structure of LSD and the neurotransmitter serotonin, an inhibitory neurotransmitter.[7] LSD apparently stimulates the same cells in the reticular formation that amphetamines activate. Disruption of serotonin neurotransmission occurs, decreasing the ability of serotonergic pathways to select the input that reaches the cortex. LSD increases the transfer of sensory information to the cortex.

Self-induced changes in neurotransmission are accompanied by enzymatic changes.[2,8] Amphetamines, for instance, block reabsorption of the neurotransmitter that may bring about an increase in the enzyme monoamine oxidase (MAO). Monoamine oxidase is responsible for breaking down the neurotransmitters. The body is attempting to bring the level of neurotransmitters back to normal. In contrast to amphetamines, the enzyme level is reduced when ingesting sedatives, such as opiates. Remember, sedatives decrease the availability of neurotransmitters in the synapse. Enzyme levels decrease in order to preserve the existing neurotransmitter.

Addiction is therefore dependent upon changes in enzyme levels. High or low levels of enzymes are experienced as craving by individuals.[7] Those who prefer relaxation will find low levels of enzymes (too much neurotransmitter) stressful, while those who seek activation, will find high levels of enzymes (too little neurotransmitter) motivating for drug use. The drug of choice is craved in order to bring the level of neurotransmitters to that reflective of arousal, sedation, or escape.

Certain genes direct the formation of particular enzymes.[9] It is believed that a given gene might influence levels of neurotransmitters through enzymatic activity such that a specific personality develops. This personality may be more susceptible to external pressures. Depending upon the sociological environment, coping styles may develop that involve pharmacological regulation of neurotransmitters and enzyme levels.

◆ CONTEMPORARY DRUGS OF CHOICE ◆

The following section examines the characteristics of various drugs including the main effects upon the central nervous system (CNS), side-effects, tolerance and withdrawal. Two main types of CNS depressants, alcohol and sedative-hypnotics, are discussed along with CNS stimulants, opioids and hallucinogens. Refer to Table 2-1 throughout this discussion. A brief look at polydrug use is included, particularly examining the phenomena of cross-tolerance and cross-dependence.

ALCOHOL

CNS Effects

Alcohol produces general depression of the CNS. The level of depression depends upon the amount consumed. Depression results from alteration of serotonin metabolism.[10] Alcohol in low dosages is often mistaken for a stimulant due to depression of the brain's inhibitory mechanisms. The cortex is susceptible to alcohol's depressant effects by way of the reticular activating system.[11] With increasing doses, the depressant effects progress down the brain stem until finally depressing the medulla oblongata. At this point, respiratory arrest occurs.[12-13]

Periods of transient amnesia or blackouts can occur during a drinking episode. During the blackout, the individual is fully conscious, but exists in a fugue-like state. The blackout may consist of total memory loss or may be fragmentary. Often the drinker remembers when prompted by others.

Neurocognitive impairments have been demonstrated in approximately 75 percent of recovering alcoholics.[14] Alcohol has a toxic effect upon the brain cells. Significant deficiencies in nutrients and thiamine also contribute to deterioration of intellectual functioning.[15] Wernicke's Syndrome results from thiamine deficiency and consists of reversible symptoms such as ataxia, confusion, loss of short-term memory, nystagmus, and blurred vision. Korsakoff's Syndrome is the later and irreversible stage of Wernicke's characterized by confabulation, inability to learn, decreased recent memory, and disorientation.

Side-Effects

There are numerous side-effects of long-term, chronic alcohol use. Alcohol acts as an irritant to the liver, gastrointestinal tract, heart and kidneys. Three distinct diseases of the liver are caused by chronic alcohol abuse. Fatty liver disease is reversible.[16] Alcoholic hepatitis is an acute disease with a mortality rate of 10 to 30 percent.[17] Cirrhosis of the liver is the most severe and is irreversible. Scar tissue produced by the cirrhosis gradually replaces the functioning liver tissue. Alcohol consumption contributes to the development of cancers of the mouth, larynx, tongue, esophagus, liver, and lung.[18] The mechanism of the carcinogenic action is unclear, but

Table 2-1
Drugs of Choice

	Sedative Hypnotics	Opioids (Narcotics)	Stimulants	Hallucinogens
Drugs	Nembutol Seconal Phenobartitol Quaaludes Valium Librium Equanil	Heroin Morphine Codeine Percodan Demerol Methadone	Benzedrine Dexedrine Desoxyn Biphetamine Ritalin Preludin Cocaine	LSD Mescaline Psilocybin Cannabis Phencyclidine (PCP)
Personality	Seeks withdrawal and relaxation	Seeks withdrawal and relaxation	Seeks activation	Seeks escape from reality
Effects	Impulsiveness Dramatic mood swings Bizarre thoughts Suicidal behavior Slurred speech Disorientation Slowed mental/ physical functioning Limited attention span	Apathy Decreased concentration and physical activity Slowed speech Drooling Itching Euphoria Nausea	Increased confidence Mood elevation Sense of energy and alertness Decreased appetite Anxiety Irritability Insomnia Transient drowsiness	Fascination with ordinary objects Heightened aestheresponse to color Vision and depth distortions Slowing of time Magnified feelings *Cannabis*: Euphoria Relaxed inhibitions Increased appetite Disorientation *PCP*: Increase BP and heart rate Paranoid thoughts and delusions
Overdose	Confusion Decreased response to pain Shallow respiration Dilated pupils Weak and rapid pulse Coma Possible death	Depressed levels of consciousness Low blood pressure Rapid heart rate Shallow breathing Convulsions Coma Possible death	Elevated BP Increased body temperature Face picking Suspiciousness Bizarre and repetitious behavior Vivid hallucinations Convulsions Possible death	Nausea and chills Increased BP, pulse and temperature Trembling Slow breathing Insomnia Dangerous behavior *Cannabis*: Panic Paranoia Fatigue Bizarre and dangerous behavior *PCP*: Violent behavior Hallucinations Delusions Coma

Table 2-1 (continued)
Drugs of Choice

	Sedative Hypnotics	Opioids (Narcotics)	Stimulants	Hallucinogens
Withdrawal	Weakness Restlessness Nausea Vomiting Headache Nightmares Irritability Depression Acute anxiety Hallucinations Seizures Possible death	Anxiety Vomiting Sneezing Diarrhea Low back pain Watery eyes Runny nose Yawning Irritability Tremors, panic Chills, sweating Cramps	Apathy General fatigue Prolonged sleep Depression Disorientation Suicidal thoughts Agitated motor activity Irritability Bizarre dreams	Not reported expect for *Cannabis*: Hyperactivity Insomnia Decreased appetite Anxiety

could be the direct result of excessive use. Alcohol, after all, damages the lining of the stomach and esophagus. Gastritis, in fact, is often the complaint that prompts initial medical attention. Alcoholics also develop pancreatitis that can result in death.[19]

Tolerance

Tolerance occurs when the amount of alcohol taken must be increased to achieve the same effects.[20] Tolerance is one sign and symptom of alcohol dependence, although there is some controversy regarding this diagnostic practice. Tolerance results due to increased metabolism of alcohol.[21] Over time, however, tolerance decreases, possibly due to a severely scarred liver that is no longer able to metabolize the alcohol.[22]

Withdrawal

Withdrawal reactions occur in those individuals who are physically dependent upon alcohol. Dependence usually develops over a period of years. The severity of the withdrawal symptoms depends upon how long the individual has been drinking and how much alcohol is typically consumed.[23] Onset of withdrawal symptoms is usually within six to twelve hours after drinking has stopped.[24] Symptoms include anxiety, agitation, irritability, tremor, diaphoresis and tachycardia. Gastrointestinal disturbances occur early during withdrawal and involve nausea, vomiting, diarrhea and anorexia. The alcoholic may also suffer from insomnia or vivid dreams. Grand mal seizures may occur within the first forty-eight hours of abstinence and are indicative of delirium tremens (DTs).

DTs are the most advanced progression of the alcohol withdrawal syndrome. An alcoholic suffering from DTs displays psychiatric symptoms of disorientation, delirium and agitation. Accompanying physical symptoms include diaphoresis, tachycardia, cardiovascular collapse and fever. Approximately 15 percent of alcoholics experiencing DTs die.[25] A history of DTs strongly indicates that future attempts at withdrawing from alcohol will produce DTs as well.

A variant of DTs is referred to as alcoholic hallucinosis. Hallucinations may be auditory, visual, olfactory or tactile and are usually seen in a patient with a relatively clear sensorium.[26] Actually, visual hallucinations occur five times more often in alcohol withdrawal than do auditory hallucinations.[15] The fact that the alcoholic can experience hallucinations, DTs, grand mal seizures, severe anxiety and hypertension indicates that the withdrawal process can be quite dangerous. Because it is impossible to predict the specific withdrawal symptoms that an alcoholic will experience, medical supervision is necessary.

SEDATIVE-HYPNOTICS

This class of drugs is the most widely prescribed group of drugs.[27] The term sedative refers to the calming effects while the word hypnotic describes the drug's ability to induce a sleep-like state. The sedative-hypnotic drugs include barbiturates (eg. amobarbital, secobarbital or phenobarbital), hypnotics (eg. placidyl, chloral hydrate, meprobamate or methaqualone), and the antianxiety agents, otherwise known as the benzodiazepines. Benzodiazepines include such drugs as diazepam (Valium), chlordiazepoxide (Librium) and flurazepam (Dalmane).

CNS Effects

Barbiturates are prescribed as sedatives, hypnotics (sleeping pills), anesthetics and anticonvulsants. The main site of action of the barbiturates is the CNS. The barbiturates depress the CNS and an overdose of this drug produces coma. All the hypnotic drugs are CNS depressants.

In terms of CNS effects of the benzodiazepines, research indicates the existence of a CNS benzodiazepine specific receptor.[28] The benzodiazepines produce their action by affecting the regulatory sites on a benzodiazepine receptor complex.[29] The benzodiazepine receptor is similar to gamma-aminobutyric acid (GABA) receptors. GABA is an important inhibitory transmitter in the CNS. Activation of the benzodiazepine receptor also produces neuronal depression.[30]

Side-Effects

The side-effects for barbiturates include drowsiness, hangover and residual effects on motor skills. Barbiturates also alter sleep stages by decreasing rapid-eye-movement (REM) sleep. When the drug is discontinued, a rebound of these sleep alterations or, in other words, an increase in the normal amount of REM sleep may occur.[27] Depression of respiration occurs with barbiturate ingestion as well.

Side-effects for the hypnotics are varied depending upon the particular drug involved. For example, placidyl produces positional nystagmus, diplopia, hangover, hypotension, nausea and vomiting. The main side-effects for meprobamate, another hypnotic, are ataxia and drowsiness. Methaqualone produces fatigue, dizziness, headache, loss of appetite, nausea and abdominal cramps.[31] Side-effects for benzodiazepines usually include drowsiness, motor incoordination, and ataxia. Some individuals experience hostility, confusion, dry mouth, blurred vision and headaches.[27]

Tolerance

For the barbiturates, tolerance develops quickly and even though increasingly higher dosages are required to achieve the same effect, the lethal dose does not increase. Unfortunately, tolerance often leads to overdose. Tolerance for most of the hypnotics resembles tolerance for barbiturates. When benzodiazepines and the other sedative-hypnotics are chronically used, not only does tolerance occur, but cross-tolerance to other CNS depressants is also involved.[27]

Withdrawal

There are similarities in the withdrawal symptoms of drugs within the CNS depressant class. Reference to this process is known as the "general depressant withdrawal syndrome."[21] The actual withdrawal varies depending upon how long the drug has been abused and the dosages consistently taken. According to Jaffe, the intensity and duration of the withdrawal syndrome is influenced by the half-life of the abused drug.[21] For example, withdrawal from short-acting drugs, such as chloral hydrate, produces intense syndromes lasting approximately five to seven days. This is contrasted to long-acting drugs, such as phenobarbital or Valium. The long-acting drugs have less intense syndromes, but tend to be more prolonged.

Withdrawal from short-acting and intermediate-acting depressants consists of anxiety, panic, weakness, orthostatic hypotension, tachycardia, fasciculation, sweating, insomnia, nausea, vomiting, diarrhea and anorexia.[21] These symptoms are the most severe during the first two to three days of withdrawal. Seizures may occur on the second or third day of withdrawal.[21] A delirium or psychosis, similar to that produced by alcohol, may develop.

The long-acting depressants have similar withdrawal symptoms including anorexia, nausea, vomiting, sweating and twitching.[32] Withdrawal symptoms that are prominent features of long-acting depressants include attacks of panic, depression, severe agitation, and anxiety.[33] These symptoms may last two to three weeks, taking four to eight days to first develop.[34] Grand mal seizures can occur on the seventh or eighth day.[33] In general, withdrawal from the CNS depressants can be life-threatening and requires medical attention.

CNS STIMULANTS

Stimulants increase cortical alertness. Electrical activity is increased throughout the brain and spinal cord. Action of dopamine and norepinephrine in specific brain areas is mimicked by the stimulants. Commonly abused stimulants include amphetamines, cocaine, caffeine and nicotine. Only cocaine and amphetamines (benzedrine, dexedrine, desoxyn, and biphetamine) are discussed in this chapter.

CNS Effects

Amphetamines produce their effects through several mechanisms. These drugs directly stimulate the adrenergic receptors.[35] Amphetamines also indirectly increase norepinephrine levels at the synapse through inhibition of the monoamine oxidase enzymes. It is also likely that the drugs inhibit the reuptake of norepinephrine, making more of the neurotransmitter available at the synapse.

Cocaine acts on the three neurotransmitters of norepinephrine, serotonin and dopamine.[36] Dopamine, however, is the neurotransmitter that is involved in the powerful reward process that facilitates cocaine's addictive properties. Dopamine-releasing neurons are important components of behavioral arousal or motivational states.[35] Cocaine seems to work at the terminal end of the neuron by prolonging dopamine's time in the synapse. Dopamine is allowed to remain with its postsynaptic receptor due to cocaine's blocking of the dopamine reuptake mechanism.[35] The behavioral result of this CNS effect is reward and euphoria.

Side-Effects

Toxic effects of low-to-moderate doses of amphetamines or cocaine are mainly exaggerations of the physiologic effects associated with their use. To be specific, low doses of amphetamines and cocaine normally produce an increase in blood pressure, a reflexive decrease in heart rate, relaxation of bronchial smooth muscle, stimulation of the bladder sphincter, and a decrease in gastrointestinal tract motility.[37] Amphetamines and cocaine increase alertness and decrease fatigue, elevate mood and produce euphoria. Activity levels are increased and physical performance of tasks may initially improve.

With the prolonged increase in alertness, sleep patterns are disturbed. Sleep disturbances continue even after discontinuation of the amphetamines or cocaine. There is a characteristic REM sleep rebound effect when the drugs are discontinued.[36] Negative effects of low doses include increased irritability, restlessness, difficulty sleeping, blurred vision and mental confusion.

Large doses of amphetamines or cocaine, taken to overcome tolerance, may cause various mental aberrations. The drug user may demonstrate repetitive grinding of teeth, touching and picking the face and extremities, performing the same task over and over, a preoccupation with one's own thought processes, suspiciousness and paranoia.[38] These symptoms indicate development of an amphetamine or cocaine psychosis. Auditory, visual, tactile and olfactory hallucinations may occur. Visual, olfactory and tactile hallucinations are more frequently seen in amphetamine and cocaine psychoses and often help to differentiate those syndromes from paranoid schizophrenia. In amphetamine or cocaine psychosis, there is no distinct thought disorder. Mood is not flat as is true of schizophrenia. Instead, mood is characterized by anxiety.

Other physiological effects of amphetamines and cocaine at high doses, in addition to the centrally mediated symptoms, include cardiovascular dysfunctions involving tachycardia, hypertension and life threatening arrhythmias. Nausea, vomiting, diarrhea and cramping are the typical gastrointestinal dysfunctions.[35]

Tolerance

Tolerance to amphetamines and cocaine develops with chronic use. The CNS stimulating effects and the appetite suppressant effects diminish over time.[39] Tolerance to the cardiac stimulant and convulsant effects of cocaine has been reported.[40] Both low and high dosages lead to tolerance. The rate at which tolerance develops is highly dependent upon the user's pattern of abuse and the specific amphetamine taken. Methamphetamine produces the highest rate of tolerance.[35]

Withdrawal

With the abrupt discontinuation of amphetamine use, no physical withdrawal symptoms are experienced. Psychological changes, however, may develop and last over a period of several months.[35] Apathy, long periods of sleeping, irritability, depression and disorientation characterize the psychological changes experienced. Paranoia usually disappears within seven to ten days, but delusions may persist for a year or longer.

The abrupt withdrawal from cocaine produces a characteristic abstinence syndrome. During withdrawal, there is a strong craving for the drug. This strong craving often prevents individuals from successfully withdrawing from the drug. The individual experiences extreme fatigue and as a result, sleeps for prolonged periods of time. Sensations of increased hunger and behavioral depression may also occur.[41]

OPIOIDS

Opioids are typically termed narcotics and include the natural drugs developed from the opium poppy as well as synthetic drugs pharmacologically similar to the natural opium products. Opioids include such drugs as opium, heroin, meperidine (Demerol), methadone, oxycodone (in Percodan), codeine, pentazocine (Talwin), propoxyphene (Darvon), etc. Each drug may produce subtle differences in terms of effects and their duration, severity of side-effects, and withdrawal. There are enough general effects, common to all, that the group of drugs can be described as a whole.

CNS Effects

All opioids affect the central nervous system by producing mood changes and mental clouding.[42] Reduction of pain and production of drowsiness are important medical effects. As the dose is increased, mental changes, drowsiness and analgesia also increase. The opioid drugs decrease response to painful stimuli by affecting the release of acetylcholine, norepinephrine and dopamine.[42] Opioids produce their effects by binding to specific receptor sites. Researchers have proposed the existence of more than one type of opioid receptor.[43] Attachment to one type of receptor produces specific effects that may be different from the effects resulting from attachment to another type of receptor.

Opioids are often classified as agonists, antagonists, or agonist-antagonist drugs.[44] Agonist opioids, such as morphine, produce both the desired and undesired drug effects. An agonist, in other words, produces a response after binding to a given receptor site. Antagonist opioids, such as noloxone (Narcan), do not produce any response after binding with the receptor site. In this case, the drug blocks the receptor from binding with other opioids.[45] Because noloxone blocks the morphine receptor sites, it is utilized to control the overdose of morphine. Noloxone prevents morphine from producing its effects.

Talwin is an example of an opioid agonist/antagonist drug, meaning that Talwin may bind with a receptor and produce effects as well as prevent other opioids, such as morphine, from reaching receptor sites. A morphine-dependent person will actually perpetuate withdrawal symptoms when taking Talwin.[46]

Side-Effects

Restriction of pupils is an effect of opioids, resulting from stimulation of the oculomotor nerve.[47] Pupillary restriction does not abate with tolerance and is one side-effect that aids in diagnosis. Opioid drugs also decrease function of the brain stem respiratory centers.[42] Constipation is produced by opioid use and prolonged drug use may result in fecal impaction. Tolerance to the constipating effects rarely develops.[48] Additionally, peripheral blood vessels are dilated with orthostatic hypotension exhibited upon standing.[49] Adverse side-effects of opioids commonly include drowsiness, nausea and vomiting. Delirium occasionally occurs.

Tolerance

Tolerance to opioids is variable and inconsistent. Tolerance may develop for certain effects, but not for others. In contrast to alcohol, tolerance to the opioids drops dramatically after a period of abstinence, and drug users are known to abstain for a while in order to bring their drug habit down to affordable levels.[42] Also, unlike barbiturates, the lethal dose of opioids increases with the advent of tolerance. Tolerance to one opioid usually extends to other opioids. In fact, signs and symptoms of withdrawal for the most part can be controlled with another opioid. Other opioids are often used in detoxifying the opioid addict.[50] When the substitute opioid is withdrawn, however, there are withdrawal symptoms characteristic of the new drug.

Withdrawal

Withdrawal severity depends upon the type and amount of the opioid used. Usually the opioids with a shorter duration of action produce more severe, but shorter withdrawal syndromes.[21] Meperidine (Demerol) is an example of a short acting opioid, thus producing withdrawal within about three hours after the last dose.[51] Morphine and closely related drugs (eg. Dilaudid, Numorphan, and heroin) produce withdrawal symptoms within 8 to 12 hours of the last dose. Methadone, on the other hand, produces withdrawal over a longer period of time. The severity of the methadone withdrawal can be perpetuated by Narcan. In general, the withdrawal from opioids is characterized by fretful sleep, gooseflesh, irritability, inability in handling minor problems, anxiety and multiple physical complaints. The physical symptoms often motivate continued use of the drug.[21]

HALLUCINOGENS

Chemicals that distort reality are commonly referred to as hallucinogens. Although this category is broad in nature, one common effect is the occurrence of hallucinations. These drugs include lysergic acid diethylamide (LSD), cannabis (marijuana), hashish, psilocybin (mushrooms), mescaline (peyote), phencyclidine (PCP) and MDA (methoxy-amphetamine).

The four drugs discussed in this chapter are LSD, mescaline, marijuana and PCP. These four drugs were chosen due to their differing chemical structures. Other hallucinogens have chemical structures similar to at least one of these four drugs. For example, LSD and psilocybin are similar structurally and, as a result, have similar effects. Mescaline has similar properties to MDA. Marijuana, hashish and hash oil all contain the psychoactive substance THC (delta-9-tetrahydrocannabinol). PCP is probably in a class by itself in terms of drug effects.

CNS Effects

The mechanism by which LSD produces its CNS effects are largely unknown. This drug possibly stimulates cells in the reticular formation in a fashion similar to amphetamines.[52] Fiber tracts utilizing serotonin are disrupted as well so that transfer of sensory information to the cortex is potentiated.

Mescaline is chemically related to the catecholamine neurotransmitters. The hallucinatory effects, however, are similar to those produced by LSD.[53] Cannabis and other drugs with THC compounds affect brain amine levels.[54] Structural changes in neurons may also occur with chronic cannabis use.[55]

PCP acts to some degree as a nonspecific CNS depressant, similar to barbiturates and alcohol. In addition to this action, PCP also functions as an anticholinergic similar to atropine, as an anesthetic, and as a psychedelic. Due to the variety of actions, it appears that PCP affects more than one neurotransmitter. In terms of chemical structure, PCP is similar to both norepinephrine and serotonin.[56] PCP possibly inhibits norepinephrine reuptake as well as reduces MAO inhibitor activity.[57] Large doses of PCP may increase brain acetylcholine levels. Increased brain acetylcoholine levels are responsible for the behavioral manifestations typical of PCP overdose.[58]

Side-Effects

Definite effects on the autonomic nervous system are produced by LSD. These effects include dizziness, hot and cold flashes, dry mouth (occasionally excessive salivation), dilated pupils, elevated body temperature and increased blood pressure.[9] This drug is abused for the experience of altered sensations; mood; abnormality of color, time and space perception; and visual hallucinations. There may be alterations in reasoning produced by LSD that lead the user to feel omnipotent or profoundly insightful.

Several adverse reactions from LSD use occur in the form of panic reactions, overt psychosis, and flashbacks.[9] Extreme anxiety or panic reactions stem from altered perception and the belief that one is unable to return from the "trip." Panic reactions are often dangerous due to the hyperactivity, labile mood and illogical reasoning that accompany the effect. The user may attempt illogical methods to escape from the trip, eg. jumping out of a window. The panic reaction may last as long as 24 to 48 hours.[59] Except for injuries produced as a result of this illogical thinking, panic reactions fortunately do not leave any residual effect.

The LSD psychosis is characterized by a true loss of touch with reality. Return to normal mental functioning may occur slowly, requiring the individual to be hospitalized for a lengthy period of time. This psychosis occurs primarily in individuals who are prepsychotic prior to drug use.[59] Flashbacks are often considered one of the most frightening adverse effects of LSD. Flashbacks are an actual recurrence of the "trip" weeks or months after the LSD has last been ingested. Schick and Smith report that flashbacks are variable and unpredictable, occurring most frequently just before going to sleep, while driving and during periods of high stress.[59] Flashbacks decrease in occurrence over time.

High doses of mescaline produce mydriasis (pupil dilation), increased heart rate and blood pressure and elevated body temperature. These symptoms result from actions on peripheral adrenergic nerve fibers.[53] Because of respiratory depression, toxic doses can lead to convulsions and death. Toxic overdose of mescaline, however, is rare due to its low potency in comparison with other hallucinogens.[53] Psychologic effects of mescaline are similar to LSD including delusions, paranoid thought patterns and panic.

The effects of cannabis have been debated over the years. Many believe that there are relatively few physiological and psychological side-effects. This is especially true of marijuana used in low doses on an infrequent basis. However, evidence now indicates that marijuana does produce cardiovascular, respiratory, neuroendocrine and nervous system effects.[60] Tachycardia and orthostatic hypotension are known to occur. Respiratory problems are associated with the inhalation of combustible products. Chronic exposure to marijuana smoke impairs pulmonary defense mechanisms. Precancerous lung tissue may develop.[61] Neuroendocrine effects of marijuana occur due to impact on hypothalamic-pituitary functioning.[62] Alterations in reproductive hormones, spermatogenesis and ovulation may result with chronic use.[62]

It still is not clear, however, whether the main effects of marijuana are temporary or, with chronic use, permanent. These main effects involve feelings of relaxation, euphoria and sensory alterations. Judgment of time and distance is impaired along with recent memory, learning ability and physical coordination.[9] High doses can produce tremors, muscle rigidity, myoclonus and organic toxicity. In terms of neurologic effects, amotivation syndrome is associated with long-term use of marijuana.[63] Amotivation syndrome is characterized by apathy, a lack of concern for the future and a loss of motivation. Marijuana also potentiates occurrence of psychiatric symptomatology in those individuals prone to these problems.

The ingestion of PCP produces myriad effects. Behavioral effects are variable and somewhat dependent upon the person and the environment. These behaviors often lead to life-threatening situations.[64] The PCP abuse syndrome is classified into four successive stages.[53] The first stage, acute PCP toxicity, is reflective of combativeness, catatonia, convulsions and coma. The severity of these symptoms are dose-related. There may be a fatal hypertensive crisis. Visual disturbances occur and typically include distortions in size and shape of objects and in distance perception. Auditory hallucinations are common. Phase I may last up to 72 hours with eventual clearing of the sensorium.

Phase II or toxic psychosis does not always follow the acute toxic phase, and when it does occur, the psychosis tends to last approximately seven days.[53] A toxic psychosis is dose-related and is more apt to occur with chronic use. The psychosis may involve both visual and auditory hallucinations, agitation, paranoid delusions, and disturbed judgment. The user is often combative and hostile, and should be considered dangerous.

Phase III of the PCP syndrome (psychotic episodes) mimics schizophrenia and may last for a month or more.[53] A thought disorder, paranoid ideation, and disturbances in affect are common. Prepsychotic individuals are more likely to exhibit these psychotic episodes.

The fourth and final phase is referred to as PCP-induced depression and is especially dangerous due to the high suicide potential. This phase may follow any of the aforementioned phases, but is most likely to occur if the user exhibited the Phase III syndrome. Often the user in Phase IV uses other street drugs to alleviate the depression. A prolonged mental dysfunction accompanies this depression, which lasts for several months.

Tolerance

Development of dependence, either physical or psychological, does not occur with LSD or mescaline use. Tolerance to LSD, however, does develop very rapidly with repeated daily doses over a three- to four-day period. Recovery from tolerance also occurs rapidly so that a chronic user can get the desired effect after a period of abstinence. Tolerance to LSD also means that the user will have tolerance for mescaline and psilocybin. Mescaline tolerance takes a longer period than does LSD tolerance to develop.

Chronic use of marijuana does lead to development of physical dependence and tolerance. Tolerance is dose specific and depends upon the pattern of use. Psychological dependence leads susceptible users to increase drug-seeking behavior. Physical dependence for PCP does not occur. Chronic users of PCP, however, develop a psychological dependence experienced as craving for the drug. Tolerance to PCP occurs as the result of daily use.

Withdrawal

Withdrawal syndromes are not reported for LSD, mescaline, and PCP due to lack of physical dependence. Withdrawal primarily consists of controlling the psychological dependence reported for PCP. Marijuana, in contrast, has a mild physical and a psychological dependence so that a slight withdrawal syndrome may be noted. This withdrawal syndrome appears within hours of the last dose. The individual may experience irritability, restlessness, anorexia, insomnia, sweating, nausea, vomiting and diarrhea.[65]

◆ POLYDRUG USE ◆

Many addicts use more than one drug. For example, cocaine users often drink alcohol to control the high experienced from the cocaine. Marijuana smokers also commonly use alcohol. Many users who inject either cocaine or other amphetamines (particularly methamphetamine), prefer the combination of effects generated by stimulants and narcotics. The brief and intense orgasmic high of the stimulant is followed by the prolonged euphoria resulting from drugs such as heroin.

Unfortunately, whenever there are two or more drugs within the body simultaneously, the potential for a drug interaction exists. Drug interactions add to the complexity of symptoms experienced. The withdrawal process becomes more difficult to manage. Polydrug use often explains why the preferred drugs given to manage abstinence syndromes fail to be effective.

Specific concepts are used to describe the type of interactions that occur with the use of multiple drugs. Drug interaction effects are commonly referred to as addition, potentiation, and inhibition. Although not specifically related to drug interaction, cross-dependence and cross-tolerance are two processes important for determining how chronic use of one drug impacts the effects of another drug within the same class.

ADDITION

When two or more drugs that produce the same effects are used together, additive effects may occur.[66] Addition occurs when the effects are greater than what would be expected if any one drug was used alone. However, the effects are merely cumulative in that the actions of the drugs are no greater than the sum results of all the drugs used.

POTENTIATION

Two drugs taken together may produce an interaction in which one drug enhances or potentiates the effects of the other drug.[66] This enhancement of effect may result from one drug changing the method in which the other drug is metabolized, absorbed or excreted.

Another type of potentiation is synergism. Synergism occurs when two or more drugs combine to create a greater effect than that which would be expected from the simple addition or combination of effects. The CNS depressant drugs produce synergistic actions that can be extremely dangerous. For example, death can occur when alcohol is combined with barbiturates, benzodiazepines or opioids.[66] Signs of synergism include decreased blood pressure, depression of respirations, staggering, excessive sedation and slurred speech. Synergism must be carefully considered when administering CNS depressants as a method of withdrawing an individual from a given drug. A person with a high blood alcohol level, for instance, may experience synergism when prescribed Librium, a common drug given during detoxification.

INHIBITION

This type of drug interaction occurs when one drug lessens or completely reverses the effects of the other drug taken in combination.[66] For example, the antibiotic tetracycline's effects are reduced when taken in combination with milk or an antacid. Additionally, barbiturates or alcohol are occasionally taken with amphetamines in order to control the anxiety produced by the CNS stimulants. Caffeine is often given by lay persons to those intoxicated with alcohol as a method of reducing the depressant effects of alcohol. Even though caffeine counteracts the depressant effects of alcohol, the symptoms related to alcohol intoxication are not affected by caffeine.

Inhibition that totally cancels out the effects of another drug is referred to as antagonism.[66] Antagonism usually occurs when two drugs with opposite pharmacologic actions are taken simultaneously. The concept of antagonism was previously discussed in reference to the opioid Narcan. Narcan blocks opioid receptors so that other opioids cannot produce the effect of respiratory depression. Narcan, as a result, is often employed in the emergency room during an opioid overdose.

CROSS-DEPENDENCE/CROSS-TOLERANCE

These drug effects occur when the dependent person tries drugs similar to the one upon which he or she is currently dependent. In order for cross-dependence and cross-tolerance to occur, the new drug taken must be from the same pharmacological class as the drug of choice.[9] Cross-tolerance refers to the likelihood that tolerance to one drug will produce tolerance to another drug in the same pharmacologic classification. In other words, tolerance to one drug results in a lessened response to another drug.[9]

Drugs from the same pharmacological class have the ability to alleviate withdrawal symptoms produced by the chronically used drug. This tendency is referred to as cross-dependence. Librium is often used during detoxification from alcohol. Librium and alcohol are both CNS depressants. Another example is morphine's ability to reduce the withdrawal discomfort of heroin. Both of these drugs are from the opioid classification.

◆ CONCLUSIONS ◆

This chapter examined the specifics of a variety of drugs. Typical styles of coping with stress may influence drug selection. Drugs in the major classifications were discussed, particularly in terms of their CNS effects, general side-effects and ability to produce tolerance and withdrawal syndromes. The major drug classes were CNS depressants (sedative-hypnotics and alcohol), CNS stimulants, opioids and hallucinogens. Polydrug use was also considered with special emphasis given to the processes of addition, potentiation and inhibition. Cross-dependence and cross-tolerance were described as involving drugs within the same pharmacological class.

References

1. Milkman H, Sunderwirth S: Addictive processes. *J Psychoactive Drugs* 14(3): 177-192, 1982.
2. Goldstein A: High on research. *J Drug Alcohol Dep* 3(3): 6-9, 1979.
3. Wikler A: Some implications of conditioning theory for problems of drug abuse. *Behav Sci* 16: 92-97, 1971.
4. Milkman H, Frosch W: The drug of choice. *Psychedelic Drugs* 9(1): 11-24, 1977.
5. Freedman R, Marwaha J: Effects of acute and chronic amphetamine treatment on Purkinje neuron discharge in rat cerebellum. *J Pharmacol Exp Ther* 212: 390-396, 1980.
6. Sorensen S, Johnson S, Greedman R: Persistent effects of amphetamine on Purkinje neurons following chronic administration. *Brain Res* 247: 365-371, 1982.
7. Sunderwirth S: Biological mechanisms: Neurotransmission and addiction. In Milkman H, Shaffer H (Eds.): *The Addictions: Multidisciplinary Perspectives and Treatments*. Lexington, MA: D.C. Heath and Company, 1985.
8. Goldstein A, Goldstein D: Enzyme expansion theory of drug tolerance and physical dependence. *Association for Research in Nervous and Mental Disease* 46: 265-267, 1968.
9. Milby J: *Addictive Behavior and Its Treatment*. New York: Springer Publishing Company, 1981.
10. Davis V, et al: The alteration of serotonin metabolism to 5-hydroxytrptophan by ethanol ingestion in man. *J Lab Clin Med* 69(1): 132-140, 1967.
11. Bluhm J: *When You Face the Chemically Dependent Patient: A Practical Guide for Nurses*. St. Louis, MO: Ishiyaku EuroAmerica, Inc., 1987.
12. Himwich H, Callison D: The effect of alcohol on evoked potentials of various parts of the central nervous system of the cat. In Kissin B & Begleiter H (Eds.): *The Biology of Alcoholism: Physiology and Behavior* (Vol. 2). New York: Plenum Press, 1972.
13. Ritchie J: The aliphatic alcohols. In Gilman AG, Goodman L, Gilman A (Eds.): *Goodman and Gilman's the Pharmacologic Basis of Therapeutics*. New York: Macmillan, 1980.
14. Butters N, Cermak L: *Alcoholic Korsakoff's Syndrome: An Information Processing Approach to Amnesia*. New York: Academic Press, 1980.
15. Victor M, Adams R: The effects of alcohol on the nervous system. *Research Publications of the Association for Research in Nervous & Mental Disease* 32: 526-573, 1953.
16. Lieber C, DeCarli L: Metabolic effects of alcohol on the liver. In Lieber C (Ed.): *Metabolic Aspects of Alcoholism*. Lancaster, England: MTP Press, 1977.
17. Lieber C: Liver disease and alcohol: Fatty liver, alcoholic hepatitis, cirrhosis and their interrelationships. *Ann NY Acad Sci* 283: 63-64, 1976.
18. Feldman J, Boxer P: Relationship of drinking to head and neck cancer. *Preventive Medicine* 8: 507-519, 1979.
19. Kraft A, Saletta J: Acute alcoholic pancreatitis: Current concepts and controversies. *Surg Annu* 8: 145-171, 1976.
20. Kissin B: Theory and practice in the treatment of alcoholism. In Kissin B & Begleiter H (Eds.): *The Biology of Alcoholism*: Vol. 5. Treatment and Rehabilitation of the Chronic Alcoholic. New York: Plenum Press, 1977, pp. 1-51.
21. Jaffe J: Drug addiction and drug abuse. In Gilman AG, Goodman L & Gilman A (Eds.): *Goodman and Gilman's the Pharmacologic Basis of Therapeutics*. New York: Macmillan, 1980, p. 551.

22. Cicero T: Tolerance to and physical dependence on alcohol: Behavioral and neurobiological mechanisms. In Lipton M, DiMascio A & Killam K (Eds.): *Psychopharmacology: A Generation of Progress*. New York: Raven Press, 1978.
23. Mello N, Mendelson J: The development of alcohol dependence: A clinical study. *McLean Hospital Journal* 1: 64-84, 1976.
24. Johnson R: The alcohol withdrawal syndromes. *Q J Stud Alcohol*, Supplement No. 1:66-76, 1961.
25. Sellers E, Kalant H: Alcohol intoxication and withdrawal. *N Engl J Med* 294(4): 757-762, 1976.
26. American Psychiatric Association: *Diagnostic and Statistical Manual of Mental Disorders*. (3rd ed. revised). Washington, DC: Author, 1987.
27. Harvey S: Hypnotics and sedatives. In Gilman AG, Goodman L & Gilman A (Eds.): *Goodman and Gilman's the Pharmacological Basis of Therapeutics*. New York: Macmillan, 1980.
28. Gavish M, Snyder S: Soluble benzodiazepine receptors: GABAergic regulation. *Life Sci* 26(8): 579-582, 1980.
29. Olsen R Leeb-Lundberg F: Convulsant and anticonvulsant drug-binding sites related to GABA-regulated chloride ion channels. *Adv Biochem Psychopharmacol* 26: 93-102, 1981.
30. Paul S, Marangos P, Skolnick P: The benzodiazepine-GABA-chloride ionophore receptor complex: Common site of minor tranquilizer action. *Biol Psychiatry* 16(3): 213-229, 1981.
31. Inaba D, Ray GR, Newmeyer JA, Whitehead C: Methaqualone abuse: Luding out. *J Am Med Assoc* 224(11): 1505-1509, 1973.
32. Hollister L, Motzenbecker F, Degan R: Withdrawal reactions from chlordiazepoxide (Librium). *Psychopharmacologia* 2: 63-68, 1961.
33. Hanna S: A case of oxazepam (Serenid D) dependence. *Br Journal Psychiatry* 120: 443-445, 1972.
34. Winokur A, Rickels K, Breenblatt DJ, Snyder PJ, Schatz NJ: Withdrawal reaction from long-term, low-dosage administration of diazepam. *Arch Gen Psych* 37: 101-105, 1980.
35. Morgan J: The clinical pharmacology of amphetamine. In Smith D (Ed.): *Amphetamine, Use, Misuse and Abuse*. Boston, MA: G.K. Hall, 1978.
36. Weiss B, Laites V: Enhancement of human performance by caffeine and the amphetamines. *Pharmacol Rev* 14: 1-36, 1967.
37. Haefely W, Bartholini G, Pletscher A: Monoaminergic drugs: General pharmacology. *Pharmacol Therapeutics* 3: 185-218, 1976.
38. Connell P: *Amphetamine Psychosis*. London: Chapman & Hall, 1958.
39. Castellani S, Ellenwood E, Kilbey M: Behavioral analysis of chronic cocaine intoxication in the cat. *Biol Psychiatry* 13: 203-206, 1978.
40. Matsuzaki M: Alteration in pattern of EEG activities and convulsant effect of cocaine following chronic administration in the rhesus monkey. *Electroencephalogr Clin Neurophysiol* 45: 1-15, 1978.
41. Post R, Kotin J, Goodwin K: The effects of cocaine on depressed patients. *Am J Psychiatry* 131: 511-517, 1974.
42. Jaffe J, Martin W: Opioid analgesics and antagonists. In Gilman AG, Goodman L, & Gilman A (Eds.): *Goodman and Gilman's the Pharmacological Basis of Therapeutics*. New York: Macmillan, 1980.
43. Martin W, Gilbert PE: The effects of morphine- and nalorphine-like drugs in the non-dependent and morphine-dependent chronic spinal dog. *J Pharmacol Exp Ther* 197(3): 517-532, 1976.
44. Fishman J, Hahn E: The opiates. In Richter R (Ed.): *Medical Aspects of Drug Abuse*. Hagerstown, MD: Harper & Row, 1975.
45. Hughes J, Kosterlitz H: Opioid peptides. *Br Med Bull* 33: 157-161, 1977.
46. Jasinski D, Martin W, Hoeldtke R: Effects of short- and long-term administration of pentazocine in man. *Clin Pharmacol Ther* 11: 385-403, 1972.
47. Lee H, Wang S: Mechanism of morphine-induced miosis in the dog. *J Pharmacol Exp Ther* 192(2): 415-431, 1975.
48. Hug C: Characteristics and theories related to acute and chronic tolerance development. In Mule S & Brill H (Eds.): *Chemical and Biological Aspects of Drug Dependence*. Cleveland, OH: CRC, 1972.
49. Alderman E, Barry WH, Graham AF, Hamson DC: Hemodynamic effects of morphine and pentazocine differ in cardiac patients. *N Engl J Med* 287(13): 623-627, 1972.
50. Ream N, et al: Opiate dependence and acute abstinence. In Richter R (Ed.): *Medical Aspects of Drug Abuse*. Hagerstown, MD: Harper & Row, 1975.
51. Isbell H, White W: Clinical characteristics of addictions. *Am J Med* 14: 558-565, 1953.
52. Dimijiam G: Contemporary drug abuse. In Goth A (Ed.): *Medical Pharmacology Principles and Concepts*. St. Louis, MO: C.V. Mosby, 1974.
53. Ray O: *Drugs, Society and Human Behavior*. St. Louis, MO: C. V. Mosby, 1978.
54. Johnson K, Dewey W: The effect of delta-9-tetrahydrocannabinol on the conversion of [3H] tryptophan to 5-[3H] hydroxytryptamine in the mouse brain. *J Pharmacol Exp Ther* 207: 140-150, 1978.

55. Myers W, Heath R: Cannabis sativa: Ultrastructural changes in organelles of neurons in brain septal region of monkeys. *J Neurol Sci* 4: 9-17, 1979.

56. O'Donnell S, Wanstall J: Actions of phencyclidine on the perfused rabbit ear. *J Pharm Pharmacol* 20(2): 125-131, 1968.

57. Usdin E, Usdin V: Effects of psychotropic compounds on enzyme system II: In vitro inhibition of monoamine oxidase. *Proceedings of the Society for Experimental Biology and Medicine* 108: 461-463, 1961.

58. Domino E, Wilson A: Psychotropic drug influences on brain acetylcholine utilization. *Psychopharmacologia* 25: 291-298, 1972.

59. Schick J, Smith D: Analysis of the LSD flashback. *J Psychedelic Drugs* 3(1): 13-19, 1970.

60. Benowitz N, Jones R: Cardiovascular effects of prolonged delta-9-tetrahydrocannabinol ingestion. *Clin Pharmacol Ther* 18(3): 287-297, 1975.

61. Leuchtenberger C, et al: Cytological and cytochemical effects of whole smoke and of the gas vapor phase from marijuana cigarettes on growth and DNA metabolism of cultured mammalian cells. In Nahas G (Ed.): *Marijuana: Chemistry, Biochemistry and Cellular Effects*. New York: Springer Verlag, 1976.

62. Smith C, Ruppert M, Beoch N: Comparison of the effects of marijuana extract and delta-9-tetrahydrocannabinol on gonadotropin levels in the rhesus monkey. *Pharmacologist* 21: 203, 1979.

63. Sharma B: Cannabis and its users in Nepal. *Br J Psychiatry* 127: 550-552, 1975.

64. Burns R, Lerner S: The causes of phencyclidine-related deaths. *Clin Toxicol* 12(4): 463-481, 1978.

65. Jones R, Benowitz N, Bachman J: Clinical studies of cannabis tolerance and dependence. *Ann NY Academy Sci* 282: 221-239, 1976.

66. Martin E: *Hazards of Medication*, 2nd ed. Philadelphia, PA: Lippincott, 1978.

The Psychodynamics
of Substance Abuse

INTRODUCTION

In this chapter, a foundation for treatment by occupational therapists is formed based on the psychodynamics of substance abuse. It is doubtful that successful recovery is truly possible if the pathological defenses used to maintain addiction are not eventually removed. As a result, there is a resurgence of interest in psychotherapy.[1]

Part of the reason for this interest is the fact that the limitations of the genetic and medical models of addiction in terms of prescribing treatment have become apparent.[2] Relapse rates for most treatment programs remain high, possibly indicating a need for alternative approaches. Alcoholics Anonymous (AA) has recovery percentages of 45 percent to 75 percent.[3] This success is attributed to the intuitive incorporation of psychodynamic understanding. Also, many substance abusers exhibit ego structural defects, such as antisocial or neurotic personalities, for which psychodynamic approaches may be helpful.[4-7]

Treatment of the substance abuser may be enhanced by incorporating the state of psychodynamic recovery into three hierarchical treatment levels.[8, 9] The three treatment levels organize intervention according to the psychodynamic responses to treatment. The concept of three treatment levels is discussed with particular concern regarding measuring the substance abuser's readiness for treatment level progression. Time, or the length of time since the last dose of the chemical and the number of weeks spent in treatment, is the primary indicator of readiness for the next treatment level.[9]

◆ GENERAL CONSIDERATIONS ◆

Psychodynamic theories explain human behavior and motivation as being controlled largely at the unconscious level. Emotions, conflicts and defense mechanisms are important in terms of the functional impact upon intrapersonal skills and interpersonal relationships.[10] It is not implied that substance abusers are the only individuals using defense mechanisms. In fact, everyone uses defense mechanisms to protect the ego from attack. The substance abuser, however, tends to over-use defense mechanisms, preventing growth of the ego. Without growth, anxiety eventually becomes intolerable. Drugs are therefore used as a method of controlling painful emotions.

Persons not addicted to drugs can also unsuccessfully utilize defense mechanisms. Rather than exhibiting addiction, these individuals may demonstrate somatic illnesses, neuroses and even psychoses. Therefore, a caveat must be considered. By recognizing the role of psychodynamics in the treatment of substance abuse, credence is not given to the concept of an "addictive personality." Personality theory of substance abuse has gone beyond the belief that there exists a single personality type prone to addiction. This chapter is not proposing that there is a single psychodynamic pattern common to alcoholism or other substance abuse disorders. Additionally, psychodynamics do not necessarily have a singular etiologic role in the development of substance abuse. Substance abuse is a multidetermined condition in which psychodynamics may play a part.[11]

Many recovering substance abusers do not receive psychodynamic-oriented therapy. Even though formal psychodynamics are not always employed, this does not mean that the substance abuser's defense mechanisms are not modified during the course of treatment. In fact, Kurtz believes that AA allows psychodynamic forces to operate on behalf of recovery instead of against recovery.[12]

Generally, clinical judgment determines the necessity of utilizing formalized psychodynamic approaches. Recovery for some substance abusers may be dependent upon *skillful* application of psychodynamic treatment approaches. Note the emphasis on the word "skillful." There are two main pitfalls that experienced therapists avoid. The therapist must not assume or imply that a deeper understanding of the self automatically reduces drug usage or increases responsible self-regulation of chemical consumption. Understanding of one's emotional weaknesses alone does not lead to a cure for substance abuse. This false assumption led in the past to dissatisfaction with psychodynamic-oriented therapy in the treatment of substance abuse.

The other therapeutic pitfall is the lack of awareness that some substance abusers cannot tolerate the uncovering inherent in psychodynamic approaches. Therapy may produce such strong anxiety that drugs are utilized by the substance abuser to avoid further painful exposure. During the early stages of recovery, the substance abuser's ego is not strong enough for in-depth personality exploration.[8, 9] The substance abuser's ego is developed by building coping abilities before uncovering techniques are implemented.

◆ PERSONALITY THEORY ◆

As a result of recognizing the multifactorial nature of substance abuse, personality theory has become more acceptable. Contemporary personality theories associate the experiences and consequences of drug taking to the underlying personality organization of the user.[11] A shift in emphasis from identifying a single addictive personality to examining relationships between inherited behavioral propensities or temperaments and the environment has occurred. Through interaction with the physical and social environments, these inherited temperaments are shaped into a developed personality.[13] There may, in fact, be personality types that are strongly linked with the risk for substance abuse and that could comprise a predisposition for substance abuse. Whether this predisposition produces the adverse outcome of addiction is dependent, however, on a variety of developmental and environmental factors.

According to Akiskal, Hischfeld and Yerevanian, the term temperament refers to genetically or constitutionally determined behavioral tendencies.[14] Character includes the experiences within the family structure. Personality embraces the two concepts of character and temperament by recognizing that both heredity and environment interact to determine an individual's psychologic and behavioral traits.

TEMPERAMENT

Buss and Plomin, in a review of genetic research, revealed that numerous behavioral processes have a strong heritable base.[15] They identified three temperament dimensions including activity level, emotionality and sociability as being present in the neonate soon after birth. Deviations in these heritable traits or temperaments can be connected to the risk for substance abuse.

Regarding the first temperament, activity level, research has consistently reported that hyperactivity in childhood is a risk factor for alcoholism and chemical dependency. De Obaldia, Parsons and Yohman and also Gomberg found that primary alcoholics were more likely to have childhood hyperactivity than were secondary alcoholics (alcoholism secondary to another diagnosis).[16, 17] Alterman, Petrarulo, Tarter and McGowan observed that familial alcoholics retrospectively reported more childhood hyperactivity than did nonfamilial alcoholics.[18] Mendelson found that hyperactive adolescents were more likely than their nonhyperactive peers to misuse alcohol and other drugs.[19]

The second heritable temperament, emotionality, is defined by Buss and Plomin as a susceptibility to become easily and intensely distressed.[15] The evidence indicates that becoming easily distressed may be associated with a vulnerability for addiction. Early on, these children demonstrate disturbances in emotional self-regulation. This psychological tendency is manifested in the specific behaviors of impulsiveness, irritability and aggressiveness.

Tarter found that primary alcoholics scored higher than late onset alcoholics on the Eysenck Personality Inventory Neuroticism Scale (EPI).[20-22] Gomberg observed that thirty-year-old alcoholics exhibited a number of neurotic propensities such as nail biting, shyness, nightmares, phobias, tantrums, tics, stuttering, thumb sucking and eating problems.[17] Several researchers determined that substance abusers are stimulus augmenters, ie. they react intensely to stimulation.[23, 24] Costello found that alcoholics scored in the direction of high emotional lability on the Sixteen Personality Factors Questionnaire.[25] Aronson and Gilbert described preadolescent sons of alcoholic fathers as having low frustration tolerance, emotional immaturity and moodiness.[26]

For the third heritable temperament, sociability, there is evidence that substance abusers deviate from population norms. Many researchers report that antisocial tendencies predate substance abuse.[27-31] These studies describe prealcoholics as social nonconformists and as having a propensity toward delinquency. Interpersonal relationships are characterized by lack of insight and empathy.[29]

CHARACTER AND PERSONALITY

According to personality theory, certain heritable temperaments are associated with vulnerability to substance abuse (Figure 3-1). However, these heritable temperaments alone are unlikely to cause substance abuse in adulthood. Intervening factors such as parental rearing style, peer affiliation, learned habit patterns of coping, and social and cultural sanctions undoubtedly play important roles in the final outcome. These temperaments are not immutable. Temperaments are modified by the physical and social environment throughout the developmental process.

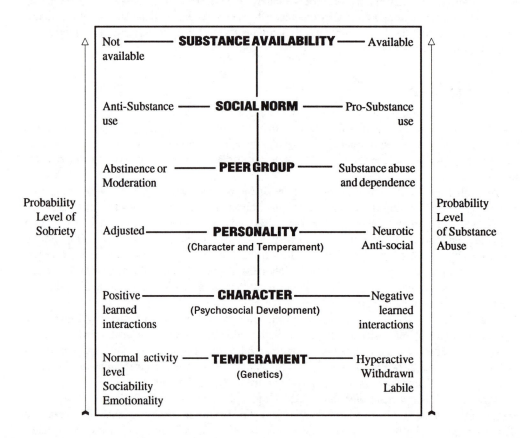

Figure 3-1. Interaction of personality with environment. *Adapted from Buss A, Plomin R: Temperament: Early Developing Personality Traits. Hillsdale, NJ: Erlbaum, 1984.*

Therefore, personality is a complex culmination of the interaction between temperaments and character. For example, the temperament of high emotionality in combination with an anxiety-producing environment (character development) could predispose someone to the personality trait of neuroticism. It follows that determining antecedent personality traits to substance abuse is ultimately dependent upon the interaction between environment and heritable temperaments.

◆ PSYCHODYNAMICS OF ADDICTION ◆

There are several psychodynamic conflicts created early in life (character development) that, if left unresolved in adulthood, could facilitate substance abuse. There is evidence that some substance abusers experience unmet dependency needs as a result of early exposure to rejection by one or both parents.[30] Overprotection of the child or the forcing of premature responsibility on the child also may contribute to adult dependency conflicts.

Overprotecting the child leads to emotional immaturity, such that the child expects others to automatically meet every desire and demand. In terms of premature responsibility, the eldest child in a substance-abusing family often experiences role reversal with the parents.[32] For example, this child assumes adult responsibility by taking care of the other children in the family as well as taking care of the using parent(s).[33] The child is so busy taking care of others that personal needs are not addressed.

Psychodynamic conflicts promoting possible substance abuse are further understood after examining the role of self-esteem in personality development.[34] Healthy self-esteem is developed from interacting with accepting parents, who are empathetic as well as worthy of admiration by the child. Given this healthy parent-child relationship, the narcissism characteristic of early childhood, transforms into a "worthwhile" self-image. Likewise, the child's idealized concept of the parent is replaced with appropriate respect and admiration for the parent.

If an adequate empathetic relationship has not been established between the parents and the child, the transformation of the narcissistic self to the worthwhile self cannot occur. Additionally, the idealized parental image is not replaced with realistic understanding of the parents. The narcissistic self is unrealistically self-sufficient and possesses abnormally high expectations of others. Not being valued by parents interferes with the ability to value the self. Adult disappointments and failures easily result due to the overly high expectations set for the self. Anger, depression, guilt and anxiety are produced, setting the stage for use of mind-altering chemicals.

Lack of internalization of parental care-taking behavior produces deficiencies in self-care involving problems in judgment and understanding consequences. There is a failure to anticipate danger that leads to a history of minor accidents, preventable medical problems, financial problems or legal difficulties.[35]

In adulthood, the individual's dependency needs cannot be met and may lead to compensatory needs for control, power and achievement. Any adult interaction that inadvertently produces the dependency conflict invokes the defense mechanisms of denial and grandiosity. Unfortunately, this grandiosity makes the adult particularly vulnerable to failure. Each failure tends to create intense feelings of fear, anger, guilt and depression, similar to the feelings experienced in childhood that were never consciously acknowledged.

Whether the adult uses alcohol or drugs to tranquilize these strong emotions depends upon the cultural environment's acceptance of alcohol or drugs. The individual must also biologically tolerate alcohol and other drugs without too many adverse side-effects. The sedative effects of alcohol and similar drugs reduce the intensity of anxiety. Once the pharmacological effects of the substance dissipate, the previous, unresolved feelings may return or may be exacerbated by further failures. Coping with substances may thus become part of a repetitive, negative cycle that if uninterrupted leads to psychological and/or physiological dependence.

The psychodynamic dependency conflict experienced by the adult is further exacerbated when drugs are used to produce feelings of increased personal power.[36] This subjective experience is particularly compelling for males who feel their masculine role is in jeopardy. In women, Wilsnack found that alcohol tends to increase feelings of femininity.[37] Alcohol and other drugs are used by both males and females as a means of compensating for feelings of inadequacy resultant from sexual role conflict.

Khantzian views decreased coping with emotions as a specific ego deficit.[35] For example, a study of 300 male substance abusers indicated that alcohol was utilized as a chemical defense against ego-threatening situations. A breakdown in the usual personality defense system made this chemical defense necessary.[38] Alcohol functioned as protection against "powerful, threatening affect states (rage, fear or helplessness); deepening despondency in depression-prone alcoholics; profound anxiety in ego-disintegration prone alcoholics; and as a means of modulating neurotic, psychotic, or sexual deviate symptomatology."[38] In fact, the study suggested that more "specificity" be introduced into the treatment of alcoholics based on the particular unconscious purpose of alcohol in defending the ego.

The main point in terms of psychodynamics is that personality may be affected by impaired character development and high risk heritable temperaments. Whether character development problems are attributed to unmet dependency needs, distortions of the self, ego deficits or jeopardized sexual roles remains to be determined. Regardless of the particular psychodynamic issue, the use of alcohol and other drugs allows the escape from intense emotions evoked by situational failures or unrealistic self-expectations.

◆ DEFENSE STRUCTURE ◆

DEFINITIONS

The concept of preferred defense structure (PDS), described by Wallace, is now introduced and is incorporated into treatment levels.[39] One of several preferred defense structures is developed and used by the substance abuser. According to Wallace, a PDS is defined as "a collection of skills or abilities, tactics and strategies, for achieving one's ends."[39] The particular PDS was learned by the substance abuser over a period of time and, as a result, has been integrated into daily modes of behavior.

As described previously, heritable temperaments and early psychodynamic factors initially played a role in the overreliance upon defense mechanisms. While actively drinking or using drugs, further modification of the PDS results. However, avoidance of strong emotions continues to dominate defense mechanism usage in adulthood.

CONFRONTATION

Many health professionals unfortunately do not recognize the substance abuser's dependence upon defense mechanisms. The professional, as a result, may inadvertently elicit transference-related behaviors in response to treatment. Douglass believed that these problems contributed to earlier assumptions that substance abusers were basically not treatable.[40]

Without full appreciation of the role of the PDS, the typical response of the health professional is to confront this defense structure. Confrontation creates intense, reactionary feelings within the substance abuser that prompt defense mechanism utilization that has been effective in the past, particularly denial, grandiosity and use of drugs to escape. It becomes difficult to stay in treatment as the urge to use drugs intensifies.

Wallace discusses the need to avoid abrupt removal of the substance abuser's PDS during the early stages of treatment.[39] Instead, the existing PDS is mobilized in order to obtain abstinence. Confrontation does occur, but only with that part of the PDS that inhibits abstinence. In other words, the substance abuser is not stripped of the only known method of coping. Total confrontation is delayed until the PDS can be replaced through treatment with alternative, more healthy coping strategies.

The following discussion explores specific aspects of the PDS. There is a review of each particular defense mechanism's function in allowing the substance abuser to avoid feelings and to continue using drugs. Implications for occupational therapy are presented in terms of paradoxically using each defense mechanism to obtain abstinence.

DENIAL

Function

Denial is the most pervasive and blatant defense mechanism employed by the substance abuser. Denial prevents problem recognition, making the voluntary seeking of treatment unlikely. Intervention is required to break through this massive denial in order that treatment may begin. Initial intervention may be conducted formally, but in most instances crisis is the precipitating factor in motivating the substance abuser to obtain help.

Actually, there is danger in viewing denial in a totally negative fashion. Many times the professional can be too hasty in confronting the denial. Often, the substance abuser is stripped of the only coping mechanism that represses strong emotions previously unrecognized. Facing strong emotions is uncomfortable, especially when alternative coping strategies are not readily available. Therefore, the substance abuser may leave treatment prematurely in order to use drugs.

Selective Denial

The substance abuser is allowed to believe for a time that most of the life problems experienced resulted from using drugs. Those problems related to immature personality development are not addressed initially. The occupational therapist carefully avoids premature uncovering by the substance abuser. Lack of well-developed coping abilities makes projective or other unstructured media inappropriate as treatment techniques during the initial stages of recovery. Structured tasks that help the substance abuser recognize current problems as a consequence of drug use are used. Later in treatment realization that not all problems are attributable to drug use occurs. By then, the substance abuser is more prepared for this revelation.

Treatment Methods

The above proposition is not to be confused with avoiding responsibility. Gradually, responsibility for obtaining abstinence is fostered as a partial solution to current situational difficulties. For example, the occupational therapist may administer an occupational history to help the substance abuser associate gradual decline in role performance with corresponding acceleration in drug use. Abstinence becomes one method for improving performance. The therapist, however, delays exploration of premorbid interpersonal problems that inhibited performance and that may be a result of ego deficits. In-depth personality exploration is more appropriate during later stages of recovery.

Denial, then, is simultaneously confronted and fostered. Denial that prevents facing the consequences of addiction is confronted. Denial that protects the immature personality is left intact so that the substance abuser can stay in treatment and begin the arduous process of developing healthier coping strategies.

PROJECTION

Function

Projection is another defense mechanism incorporated in the PDS.[39] Feelings are avoided by attributing them to others. Excuses regarding the need to use drugs are also maintained through the process of projection. Misperception of how others feel about the substance abuser may lead to episodes of drug usage. Family members are often bewildered by this behavior or may even take on the feelings that are erroneously attributed to them rather than to the substance abuser. The substance abuser, for instance, accuses his wife of being angry when really he is angry about events experienced during the day. Upon accusation, the wife eventually does become angry. Later, she is often unable to describe reasons for her strong emotions.

Occupational therapists encourage the substance abuser to explore these misperceptions regarding the feelings of others. This, however, is a slow process and must be handled expertly. There is a continuous caveat running through the procedure. Uncovering too quickly leads to exposure that often cannot be tolerated. Use of inappropriate defense mechanisms may intensify along with the urge to use drugs. The therapist's aim is not to promote understanding of projection, but to teach the substance abuser to test out what is thought about a person's feelings before formulating conclusions.

Assimilative Projection

As with denial, there is an aspect of projection that is used in therapy to mobilize abstinence. Wallace calls this assimilative projection.[39] This means that the substance abuser believes that he or she is like other substance abusers, having similar feelings and experiences. Finding out that others face the same kinds of predicaments brings a sense of relief.

Treatment Methods

Occupational therapists capitalize on assimilative projection by planning group activities that foster trust and mutual sharing. During the beginning stages of recovery, competitive activities are avoided. The substance abuser is extremely sensitive to failure or experiences that produce low self-esteem. Competition may inadvertently elicit the grandiose or exaggerated self-sufficiency as compensation mechanisms for the perceived threats to self-esteem.

Enhancing trust and mutual respect also meets any unresolved dependency needs. Often, substance abusers can become overly dependent upon fellow substance abusers who are also in treatment. The occupational therapist prevents this overly dependent behavior by facilitating independent decision-making by the substance abuser. However, getting help from others experiencing similar problems is an important aspect of initial recovery and is implemented as a treatment tool by the occupational therapist.

RATIONALIZATION

Function

Another aspect of the PDS, according to Wallace, is rationalization.[39] Rationalizations provide the substance abuser with seemingly logical reasons for drug use and are exceptionally resistant to confrontation. Blume states that the function of rationalization is to aid the substance abuser in avoiding painful reality.[41] The occupational therapist keeps in mind that reality, if faced too soon, can intensify urges to use drugs and can produce a relapse into old behavioral patterns.

Sober Rationalization

Rationalization is utilized by the therapist as a tool to maintain sobriety. When used in this manner, rationalization is referred to as sober rationalization.[39] Rationalization actually helps the substance abuser avoid pain until adequately prepared for these strong emotions. In a way, the substance abuser rationalizes reasons to stay sober. The substance abuser believes for a time that sobriety is necessary to avoid being fired or to prevent divorce.

Treatment Methods

In the beginning stages of treatment, the occupational therapist employs sober rationalization.[39] The substance abuser learns to associate role performance problems with abusive drinking or drug use. Initially, it is more likely that the substance abuser will commit to improving such difficulties as poor job performance, school failure or social problems than to working through the major issues of addiction.

A distinction is made at this point. It is possible for the substance abuser to become overinvolved with sociocultural issues. The occupational therapist guards against the substance abuser blaming drug use upon various problems. Treatment emphasizes a causal relationship between drug use and resultant role impairments. The reverse relationship, role impairment producing drug use, is not discussed or allowed as a treatment focus. Rationalization is mobilized to produce abstinence. It is not tolerated as a method to escape responsibility or the consequences of previous abusive drinking and excessive drug use.

DICHOTOMOUS THINKING

Function

The substance abuser probably grew up with parents who displayed chaotic behaviors as a result of their own substance abuse. Consequently, the addict learned to compensate for uncertainty by preferring predictability. Being intolerant of the "gray areas," tends to restrict alternatives available in problem-solving such that judgmental attitudes result.[39] The occupational therapist accommodates this desire for predictability in the early stages of treatment by providing a unit schedule, structured groups, well-planned individual sessions and organized social situations. Too much unstructured time may inadvertently produce old patterns of behavior, including inappropriate reliance upon defense mechanisms and strong urges to use drugs.

Common Dichotomies

There are many dichotomies that can surface throughout the treatment process.[42] The therapist is aware of the tendency for "all-or-none" thinking and assists the substance abuser in behaviorally working toward the "middle ground." This preference for dichotomous thinking often manifests itself as avoiding responsibility through excessive focusing on financial or marital problems. To the opposite extreme are those substance abusers who face guilt too quickly, perhaps as a result of treatment approaches that promote premature self-disclosure. Guilt may overwhelm, leading the substance abuser to leave treatment early due to difficulty coping with intense emotions. On the other hand, failure to accept a normal amount of guilt is problematic also because of too great an emphasis upon the disease concept of substance abuse.

The key to recognizing dichotomous thinking is awareness of extreme fluctuations in behavior or attitude. For example, the substance abuser may engage in excessive self-blame at one point and at another time may blame others for perceived misfortunes. Rules may be rebelled against and then the substance abuser may demonstrate overly compliant behaviors. Fluctuations may occur between impulsively expressing feelings and repressing feelings. The substance abuser may alternate between focusing obsessively on the past and refusing to discuss the past. At times, the substance abuser may be overly dependent upon staff and peers and then may refuse help. Compulsive socializing behavior may be punctuated by periods of withdrawn behavior. Exhibiting narcissism or focusing totally on others and acting either pessimistic or overly optimistic are other dichotomies that commonly occur.

Treatment Methods

The occupational therapist promotes safe exploration of behaviors that are a compromise between the two extremes inherent in dichotomies. The behavioral repertoire of the substance abuser is thus expanded so that new, more appropriate responses to everyday situations occur. In an occupational therapy group, for example, the substance abuser might exhibit too much perfectionist behavior, paying attention to detail on a craft project. During the next session, however, this perfectionism is replaced by sloppy, careless work with the substance abuser proceeding hurriedly through each craft step.

In the early stages of recovery, the therapist assists the substance abuser in deciding when imperfections are to be tolerated and when they are not acceptable. Only in the later stages of treatment are in-depth examinations of these dichotomous behaviors helpful. The goal eventually is to increase understanding of how complex issues and feelings have been successfully avoided through the use of dichotomous thinking.

OTHER DEFENSE MECHANISMS

Conflict Minimization

Wallace describes other patterns of behavior that form the core of the PDS.[39] Generally, most substance abusers do not like interpersonal conflict. This is consistent with substance abusers having difficulty coping with strong emotions. In fact, it seems that substance abusers do not do well with competitive relationships and much prefer complimentary relationships. Conflict is either minimized or avoided altogether. Obviously, this presents real challenges in therapy. Angry and hostile confrontation by the therapist is rarely successful. Actually, any confrontation, regardless of the stage of recovery, must be handled skillfully by the therapist. Extreme caution has to be exercised when using group members to confront a specific individual. The ability of the substance abuser to effectively deal with confrontation improves as alternate coping skills develop.

Passivity

Another behavior pattern commonly exhibited by the substance abuser is passivity. This seems contradictory at first, knowing that many intoxicated individuals often appear aggressive and hostile. This passivity is understood when thinking about the typical results of assertion. Often assertion or other means of active coping bring a person into normal conflict with others. Remembering that substance abusers often avoid conflict makes this passivity a logical behavior pattern. Passivity aids the substance abuser in staying away from competition and other types of win/lose outcomes. Losing facilitates usage of defense mechanisms, particularly grandiosity, denial and abusing substances.

Obsession

Along with this passivity and conflict avoidance, substance abusers are intensely focused, often to the obsessive level. Obviously, drugs are an obsession, but other obsessions may coexist with the addiction to chemicals. Substance abusers may exhibit obsessional thinking related to work, money, success, sexuality, etc. Additionally, substance abusers are highly activated, often to the point of being hyperactive. Therefore, the key in therapy is devising methods to redirect this energy, especially when lowering the level of activation is not possible. It is preferable for the substance abuser to be obsessed with sobriety and AA/NA than to be obsessed with drugs and alcohol.

Selective Attention

Similar to obsessional focusing is the substance abuser's propensity to view situations from a single, narrow perspective. In other words, substance abusers selectively attend to self-relevant information. Information not pertinent to the self is screened out, ignored or distorted in order to fit the preferred self-image. This perceptual style is directly linked with chronic low self-esteem. In therapy, the goal is not for the substance abuser to discover the "truth" about the self, but is centralized around the timing and frequency of self-discoveries.

Nonanalytical Mode of Perceiving

Given this obsessive, self-centered style of interaction, it is no surprise that many substance abusers respond to leadership styles that are charismatic, inspirational, and spiritual. A greater response is likely to emotional, persuasive appeals than to more rational approaches. The founders of AA understood this behavioral style and capitalized upon it in the design of the AA recovery process. Alcoholics Anonymous meetings are characterized by their flamboyant, emotional strategies and dynamic sharing of personal substance abusing experiences.

◆ TREATMENT LEVELS ◆

Substance abuse treatment is designed to mobilize initially the PDS status of the addicted individual. However, recovery eventually requires that the PDS be replaced with more healthy ways of coping. With this goal in mind, three treatment levels are proposed that correspond to changes in the PDS of addicted individuals that occur with ongoing intervention. Table 3-1 outlines the three treatment levels, the PDS status, the corresponding therapy issues, and the role of the substance abuser, family, and treatment team at each level. The specific role of the occupational therapist at each level is not discussed in this chapter, but is examined later in Chapters 5-7.

Table 3-1
Relationship of Treatment Level to Treatment Setting and Roles

TREATMENT LEVELS		TREATMENT SETTING	ROLE IN TREATMENT		
PDS Status	Treatment Issue		Substance Abuser	Family	Treatment Team
Mobilized ①	Loss of Control	Inpatient or Outpatient	Accept external control	Attend ALANON Attend alcohol/drug education Support need for treatment	Detoxification Alcohol/drug education Nutritional management Provide antabuse Enforce attendance to AA/Alanon (NA) Implement therapeutic milieu; provide rest Provide directive psychotherapy
Weakened ②	Coping	Inpatient or Outpatient	Develop internal control	Attend ALANON Interact in supportive family therapy	Provide directive and supportive psychotherapy Encourage attendance in AA/Alanon (NA) Continue therapeutic milieu Provide supportive family therapy
Confronted ③	Insight	Outpatient or Extended Inpatient	Relate maturely	Attend ALANON Interact in psychodynamic family therapy	Provide psychodynamic psychotherapy Support AA/Alanon (NA) Provide psychodynamic family therapy

TREATMENT LEVEL ONE

Measurement

Because there is no precise way to measure when a patient is considered to be at level one, the detoxification process is closely associated with this treatment stage. The first level of treatment is usually provided on an inpatient basis. However, treatment is gradually shifting to outpatient settings with only complicated detoxification cases (multiple drug use or dual diagnoses) admitted to an inpatient facility.

PDS Status

Regardless of treatment site at level one, the focus of intervention is on abstinence. The substance abuser's role in treatment is one of accepting external control in order to obtain sobriety. The substance abuser's loss of control over drinking or drug use indicates the need for help in achieving abstinence. External control is provided jointly by the family and treatment team. As emphasized earlier, the PDS is in full operation during this initial stage of treatment. Therefore, the PDS is not challenged, but is mobilized to assist in maintaining abstinence.

Treatment Team

Techniques of external control implemented by the treatment team usually include managed detoxification, alcohol/drug education, nutrition, rest, antabuse, directive psychotherapy, AA/NA and the treatment milieu.[8] The treatment milieu is important in terms of providing a daily imposed structure, complete with behavioral expectations. Access to alcohol and drugs is restricted, thereby removing temptations. The decision making process of determining whether to use drugs is taken away as well. The substance abuser has abdicated this decision making responsibility during treatment level one.

Family

The family's need to exercise external control varies. The family or significant others, such as employers, provide more control if detoxification is managed on an outpatient basis. For instance, the alcoholic may be required to report to the employer to take Antabuse before starting work each day. Need for the family to provide control is less when the substance abuser is treated in an inpatient program. In this situation, the family supports treatment by offering consequences if the substance abuser leaves treatment prematurely. The family has to be prepared to administer these consequences (eg. "you can't live with us"). The consequences cannot be delivered as an idle threat. Secondly, the family demonstrates their seriousness by involving themselves in Alanon and other alcohol/drug education programs offered by the treatment facility.

PDS Mobilization

External control provided by the treatment team or the family accomplishes several objectives. Mobilization of the PDS is begun by encouraging the process of assimilative projection, allowing denial of ego deficits, rationalizing sobriety and satisfying the desire for predictability. Obsessive thinking is redirected toward abstinence by emphasizing sobriety's self-relevance. Dependency needs are met. In general, self-esteem is promoted in a way that gives the substance abuser hope for the future. A specific behavior, sobriety, is provided that changes the substance abuser's life in a desired direction.

TREATMENT LEVEL TWO

Measurement

Treatment level two develops healthy coping strategies that have the potential of replacing the over-reliance upon defense mechanisms. Again, because there is no precise way of measuring when a substance abuser is ready for a specific level of intervention, level two is appropriate for substance abusers who have completed the detoxification process.[8] Generally, after two weeks of inpatient therapy or a comparable period of outpatient therapy, the substance abuser is ready for this treatment focus. Complications may prevent advancement to this treatment level and the following third level. For example, long-term use of alcohol and other drugs may produce permanent brain damage resulting in organic brain disorders. Cognitive deficits may be so severe that other therapeutic approaches are required.

PDS Status

The status of the PDS at level two is one of a weakened state. At level two, the substance abuser develops alternative, healthy coping strategies, such as expressing emotions assertively, seeking help when needed, and using relaxation techniques to control tension. Eventually, the substance abuser prefers using these coping strategies rather than drinking or using drugs to contend with complex, emotional situations. The external control provided by the treatment team and the family is gradually replaced by the substance abuser's newly emerging ability to maintain abstinence through internal control or self-discipline.

Treatment Team and Family

This shift to internal control is exemplified by the treatment team's switch from employing directive psychotherapy to providing supportive psychotherapy and cognitive/behavioral strategies.[8] The substance abuser continues involvement in AA/NA while the family remains active in Alanon. Family therapy is begun at this level with emphasis upon supportive approaches and implementation of healthy coping strategies to resolve family conflicts. Also, the substance abuser assumes an active role in the treatment milieu in order to "try on" new, healthy behaviors.

TREATMENT LEVEL THREE

Measurement

Stimulating the substance abuser's level of insight into the issues of addiction is the appropriate intervention at level three. Similar to the other levels, a general time frame can guide the decision to implement level three approaches. After completing a traditional 28-day inpatient treatment program or a comparable length of time spent in an outpatient program, the substance abuser is probably ready for insight development, given that cognitive abilities are intact.[8] Level three intervention usually occurs on an outpatient basis if the inpatient treatment was successful, or in an extended treatment situation if more intensive therapy is required. Rarely is the substance abuser ready for these intensive approaches during the initial inpatient hospitalization.

PDS Status

The status of the PDS at level three is referred to as "confronted."[43] This thorough confrontation helps the substance abuser voluntarily give up old patterns of behavior involving overreliance upon maladaptive defense mechanisms. Long-term sobriety is threatened if the substance abuser does not replace the PDS with healthy coping strategies. Recidivism may be higher for those treatment programs that do not include this type of intervention than for those programs that do include this aspect.[44]

Treatment Team and Family

Generally, at level three, the substance abuser's role in treatment is to relate to others maturely and to begin the process of introspection. Because insight is a treatment goal, family therapy is more psychodynamically-oriented as is the substance abuser's individual and group psychotherapy.[8] The substance abuser continues to attend AA/NA and the family remains in Alanon. Eventually, the substance abuser assumes a leadership role as does the family in these self-help programs.

◆ CONCLUSIONS ◆

The occupational therapist must understand the role that the PDS appears to play in treatment. These preferred behavioral strategies have been employed by the substance abuser for many years as a method of avoiding emotional pain. It stands to reason that a style of behavior cannot be challenged effectively until an alternative way of acting can be learned and integrated. Only that part of the PDS interfering with abstinence is removed during the beginning stages of treatment. Defenses are left intact initially in order to protect the substance abuser's ego and to control urges to use drugs. Premature confrontation results in a therapeutic disaster. Therapy's challenge is to use the PDS as a part of recovery.

During the early stages of recovery, the occupational therapist does not expose the preferred defense structure. The PDS is utilized to help achieve sobriety. Denial regarding the effects of substance abuse is confronted. Denying premorbid interpersonal problems is acceptable. Rationalizing reasons to use drugs is challenged, whereas rationalizing reasons to stay sober is encouraged. Projecting feelings onto others is extinguished, but believing other substance abusers have the same problems and feelings is reinforced. Obsessions are redirected from drugs to sobriety and healthy coping strategies. High levels of activation are captured by charismatic therapy programs that focus excitement on a sober future. Avoidance of conflict through passivity and minimization is managed through activities that engender trust of others. Selective self-relevant attention is utilized by making sobriety a highly individual matter that is important to one's self-image.

At the essence of this approach during the beginning stages of treatment is a respect for the learned coping strategies of the substance abuser. However, to maintain sobriety, once achieved, these coping strategies are replaced with a more open, nondefensive and authentic way of relating with others. To progress, the occupational therapist manipulates the therapeutic approach. It is with this goal in mind that therapy levels are designed.

Three treatment levels are proposed that correspond with the substance abuser's ability to control drug usage. Treatment efforts at the first level produce abstinence from drugs. An external source of control is provided that mobilizes the substance abuser's PDS. Level two approaches teach coping strategies that weaken the PDS. At level three, insight that effectively confronts the PDS is stimulated. Obviously, identifying the stage of recovery that a substance abuser has entered will indicate the appropriate treatment.

References

1. Kaufman E, McNaul JP: Recent developments in understanding and treating drug abuse and dependence. *Hosp Community Psychiatry* 43(3): 223-236, 1992.
2. Peele S: The implications and limitations of genetic models of alcoholism and other addictions. *J Stud Alcohol* 47: 63-73, 1986.
3. Leach B, Norris FL: Factors in the development of Alcoholics Anonymous (A.A.). In Kissin B & Begleiter H (Eds.): *Treatment and rehabilitation of the chronic alcoholic*. New York: Plenum Press, 1977, pp. 441-544.
4. Rounsaville BJ, Glazer W, Wilber CH, et al: Short-term interpersonal psychotherapy in methadone-maintained opiate addicts. *Arch Gen Psychiatr* 40: 629-636, 1983.
5. Woody GE, McLellan AT, Lubursky L, et al: Psychiatric severity as a predictor of benefits from psychotherapy. *Am J Psychiatry* 141: 1172-1177, 1984.
6. Rounsaville BJ, Kleber HD: Psychotherapy-counseling for opiate addicts: Strategies for use in different treatment settings. *Int J Addict* 20: 869-896, 1985.
7. Woody GE, McLellan AT, Lubursky L, et al: Psychotherapy for substance abuse. *Psychiatr Clinic North Am* 9: 547-562, 1986.
8. Zimberg S: Principles of alcoholism psychotherapy. In Zimberg S, Wallace J, & Blume SB (Eds.): *Practical Approaches to Alcoholism Psychotherapy* (2nd ed.). New York: Plenum Press, 1985, pp. 3-21.

9. Okpatu SO: Psychoanalytically oriented psychotherapy of substance abuse. *Adv Alcohol Subst Abuse* 6: 17-33, 1986.

10. Blum E: Psychoanalytic views of alcoholism: A review. *Q J Stud Alcohol* 27: 259, 1966.

11. Treece C, Khantzian E: Psychodynamic factors in the development of drug dependence. *Psychiatr Clinic North Am* 9: 399-412, 1986.

12. Kurtz E: *Not God—A History of Alcoholics Anonymous*. Center City, MN: Hazelden Foundation, 1979.

13. Tarter RE: Are there inherited behavioral traits that predispose to substance abuse? *J Consult Clin Psychol* 56(2): 189-196, 1988.

14. Akiskal S, Hirschfeld R, Yerevanian BI: The relationship of personality disorders to affective disorders. *Arch Gen Psychiatry* 40: 801-809, 1983.

15. Buss A, Plomin R: *Temperament: Early Developing Personality Traits*. Hillsdale, NJ: Erlbaum, 1984.

16. De Obaldia R, Parsons O, Yohman R: Minimal brain dysfunction symptoms claimed by primary and secondary alcoholics: Relation to cognitive functioning. *Int J Neurosci* 20: 173-182, 1983.

17. Gomberg E: The young male alcoholic. A pilot study. *J Stud Alcohol* 43: 683-700, 1982.

18. Alterman A, Petrarulo E, Tarter R, McGowan JR: Hyperactivity and alcoholism: Familial and behavioral correlates. *Addict Behav* 7: 413-421, 1982.

19. Mendelson J: Biochemical mechanisms of alcohol addiction. In Kissin B Begleiter H (Eds.): *The Biology of Alcoholism: Biochemistry* (Vol. 1). New York: Plenum Press, 1971.

20. Tarter R: Psychosocial history, minimal brain dysfunction and differential drinking patterns of male alcoholics. *J Clin Psychology* 38: 867-873, 1982.

21. Eysenck H: *The Biological Basis of Personality*. Springfield, IL: Thomas, 1967.

22. Eysenck H: Neurotic conditions. In Tarter R (Ed.): *The Child at Psychiatric Risk*. New York: Oxford University Press, 1983, pp. 245-285.

23. Sher KJ, Levenson RW: Risk for alcoholism and individual differences in the stress-response-dampening effect of alcohol. *J Abnorm Psychol* 91: 350-368, 1982.

24. Barnes G: Clinical and prealcoholic personality characteristics. In Kissin B & Begleiter H (Eds.): *The Pathogenesis of Alcoholism* (vol. 6). New York: Plenum Press, 1983, pp. 113-195.

25. Costello RM: Alcoholism and the "alcoholic" personality. In NIAAA Research Monograph No. 5: *Evaluation of the Alcoholic: Implications for Research, Theory, and Treatment*. Rockville, MD: NIAAA, 1981.

26. Aronson H, Gilbert A: Preadolescent sons of male alcoholics. *Arch Gen Psychiatry* 8: 47-53, 1963.

27. Zucker RA, Gomberg EL: Etiology of alcoholism reconsidered. *Am Psychol* 41(7): 783-793, 1986.

28. Berry J: Antecedents of schizophrenia, impulsive character, and alcoholism in males. *Dissertation Abstracts* 28: B-2134, 1967.

29. Jones M: Personality correlates and antecedents of drinking patterns in adult males. *J Consult Clin Psychol* 32: 2-12, 1968.

30. McCord W, McCord J: *Origins of Alcoholism*. Stanford, CA: Stanford University Press, 1960.

31. Robins L: *Deviant Children Grown Up: A Sociological and Psychiatric Study of Sociopathic Personality*. Baltimore, MD: Williams & Wilkins, 1966.

32. Fox R: *The Effect of Alcoholism on Children*. New York: National Council on Alcoholism, 1972.

33. Cork MR: *The Forgotten Children*. Toronto, Canada: Paperjacks, in association with Addiction Research Foundation, 1969.

34. Kohut H: *The Analysis of the Self*. New York: International Universities Press, 1971.

35. Khantzian EJ: The self-medication hypothesis of addictive disorders: Focus on heroin and cocaine dependence. *Am J Psychiatry* 142: 1259-1264, 1985.

36. McClelland DC, Davis W, Kalin R, Wanner E: *The Drinking Man*. New York: Free Press, 1972.

37. Wilsnack S: Sex-role identity in female alcoholics. *J Abnorm Psychol* 82: 253-261, 1973.

38. DeVito RA, Flaherty LA, Mozdzierz GJ: Toward a psychodynamic theory of alcoholism. *Dis Nerv System* 31(1): 43-49, 1970.

39. Wallace J: Working with the preferred defense structure of the recovering alcoholic. In Zimberg S, Wallace J & Blume SB (Eds.): *Practical Approaches to Alcoholism Psychotherapy*, 2d ed. New York: Plenum Press, 1985, pp. 23-36.

40. Douglas DB: Who is a real alcoholic? Practical help in managing alcoholism. *NY State J Med* 76: 603-607, 1976.

41. Blume EM: Psychoanalytic views of alcoholism: A review. *Q J Stud Alcohol* 27: 259-299, 1966.

42. Wallace J: Critical issues in alcoholism therapy. In Zimberg S, Wallace J & Blume SB (Eds.): *Practical Approaches to Alcoholism Psychotherapy*, 2d ed. New York: Plenum Press, 1985, pp, 37-52.

43. Moyers PA: An organizational framework for occupational therapy in the treatment of alcoholism. *Occ Th MH* 8(2): 27-46, 1988.

44. Royce JE: *Alcohol Problems and Alcoholism: A Comprehensive Survey*. New York: Macmillan, 1981.

Clinical Reasoning
and Substance Abuse

INTRODUCTION

This chapter examines the clinical reasoning process applicable to substance abusers. According to Rogers and Holm, "Clinical reasoning refers to the cognitive operations that underlie the OT process."[1] Mattingly further defines clinical reasoning as necessary for determining "the nature of a patient/client's functional status" and for inferring from this assessment "the most suitable treatment plan."[2] Clinical reasoning takes into consideration the meaning of the illness or disability as experienced by the patient or client. In this chapter, clinical reasoning is seen as a matching process that selects the best treatment for each individual substance abuser that is unique to the particular circumstances involved.

Within the literature, there is widespread support for matching the individual substance abuser with optimal treatment approaches.[3-9] This matching process is sometimes referred to as prescriptive or differential treatment. According to Finney and Moos, there are four important conceptual issues or questions inherent in matching substance abusers with treatments.[10] The questions are as follows:

1. What characteristics of the substance abuser are pertinent to the treatment selection process?
2. What treatment variables interact with the identified characteristics of the substance abuser?
3. What is the anticipated outcome of this interaction (or match) between treatment variables and the characteristics of the substance abuser?
4. When should these matching decisions be made?

The three treatment levels, discussed in Chapter 3, are an organizing framework for occupational therapy. One of the framework's purposes is to assist in selecting the most applicable occupational therapy or psychosocial frame of reference that ultimately guides the patient's evaluation, treatment planning, treatment implementation and treatment evaluation processes. Thus, the best match between the substance abuser and the appropriate treatment is achieved.

Matching considers the substance abuser's PDS status. Choice of frame of reference is therefore based upon the current treatment issue, ie. whether the substance abuser requires external control in order to attain abstinence (level one), the teaching of coping strategies in order to promote internal control (level two), or the stimulation of insight in order to foster personality development (level three).[11]

The therapeutic procedures described in this chapter are applicable to a variety of treatment settings, including inpatient and outpatient programs. The concept of three hierarchical treatment levels, designed to correspond with progressive changes in the substance abuser's preferred defense structure (PDS), is a critical factor in guiding the matching decision. Refer to Figure 4-1 and Table 4-1 to clarify the following discussion.

◆ PERTINENT SUBSTANCE ABUSER CHARACTERISTICS ◆

What characteristics of the substance abuser are pertinent in the treatment selection process?

PDS VARIABLES

Characteristics of the substance abuser are referred to as PDS variables. PDS variables include the three main treatment issues of needing external control, internal control or insight. These issues are operationally defined in terms of the substance abuser's strengths and weaknesses. For example, the substance abuser might describe a loss of control over drinking, indicating that external control is the current treatment issue.

In terms of internal control, the substance abuser might describe inability in staying sober unless others provide assistance and that daily problems create strong urges to use drugs. Indicative of the next treatment level, the substance abuser implements coping strategies to control urges to use drugs, but cannot discuss unresolved conflicts that contribute to the desire to use. In this example, the substance abuser's treatment issue revolves around development of insight.

PROBLEM CLASSIFICATION

The substance abuser also exhibits specific problems that underlie the major issues reflective of each treatment level. According to the second edition of Uniform Terminology, these

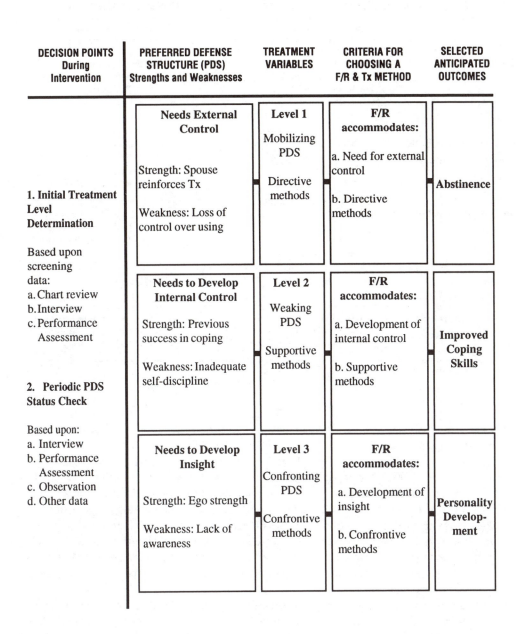

DECISION POINTS During Intervention	PREFERRED DEFENSE STRUCTURE (PDS) Strengths and Weaknesses	TREATMENT VARIABLES	CRITERIA FOR CHOOSING A F/R & Tx METHOD	SELECTED ANTICIPATED OUTCOMES
1. Initial Treatment Level Determination Based upon screening data: a. Chart review b. Interview c. Performance Assessment **2. Periodic PDS Status Check** Based upon: a. Interview b. Performance Assessment c. Observation d. Other data	**Needs External Control** Strength: Spouse reinforces Tx Weakness: Loss of control over using	**Level 1** Mobilizing PDS Directive methods	**F/R accommodates:** a. Need for external control b. Directive methods	**Abstinence**
	Needs to Develop Internal Control Strength: Previous success in coping Weakness: Inadequate self-discipline	**Level 2** Weaking PDS Supportive methods	**F/R accommodates:** a. Development of internal control b. Supportive methods	**Improved Coping Skills**
	Needs to Develop Insight Strength: Ego strength Weakness: Lack of awareness	**Level 3** Confronting PDS Confrontive methods	**F/R accommodates:** a. Development of insight b. Confrontive methods	**Personality Develop- ment**

Figure 4-1. Selecting a frame of reference for the substance abuser. Begin at lowest level with the most problems. PDS=Preferred Defense Structure; Tx=Treatment; F/R=Frame of Reference.

Table 4-1
Frame of Reference Selection and Treatment Levels

	Initial Treatment Level Determination	Periodic PDS Status Evaluation
Data Source	Screening Data: a. Chart review b. Interview c. Performance assessment	Screening Data: a. Interview b. Performance assessment c. Observation d. Other data
Characteristics of the Substance Abuser	PDS Variables: a. Strengths b. Weaknesses	New PDS Variables: a. New strengths b. Different weaknesses c. Resolved problems
Treatment Variables	PDS Status: a. Level one b. Level two c. Level three	Change in PDS Status: a. Higher level (Progress) b. Lower level (Regress)
Timing of Matching Decisions	Upon referral	PDS status change
F/R Determination (Treatment Approach)	Select one F/R based upon: a. PDS variables b. PDS status	Select New F/R or Continue: a. New PDS variables b. New PDS status

PDS = Preferred Defense Structure; F/R = Frame of Reference.

problems are characterized as occupational component dysfunctions or as occupational performance dysfunctions.[12] Refer to Figure 4-2 for clarification.

At treatment level one, these problems can be broadly categorized as cognitive (ie. orientation, level of arousal, recognition, attention span and memory), sensorimotor, socialization (ie. social conduct or ability to converse with others) or psychological (initiation and termination of activity). Sensorimotor skills are composed of neuromuscular functions (ie. reflexes, range of motion, muscle tone, strength, endurance, postural control and soft tissue integrity), sensory integration (ie. sensory awareness, sensory processing and perceptual skills) and motor functions (activity tolerance, gross and fine motor coordination, crossing the midline, laterality, etc.).[12] These classifications represent the performance components necessary for occupational functioning.[12]

At treatment level one, psychological functioning is stabilized and socialization occurs in a safe environment in order to facilitate assimilative projection. Activities of daily living skills are the occupational performance areas of concern at treatment level one. Activities of daily living skills include aspects of self-care such as feeding, toileting, grooming, dressing and hygiene.

Treatment level two focuses on a different set of problems. Advancement of the substance abuser to this treatment level means that the sensorimotor deficits and most of the cognitive deficits have been resolved. If this is not the case, it is doubtful that the substance abuser is ready for this treatment level. The remaining cognitive problems requiring treatment include aspects of cognitive integration: particularly, generalization, discrimination and problem solving. Psycho-

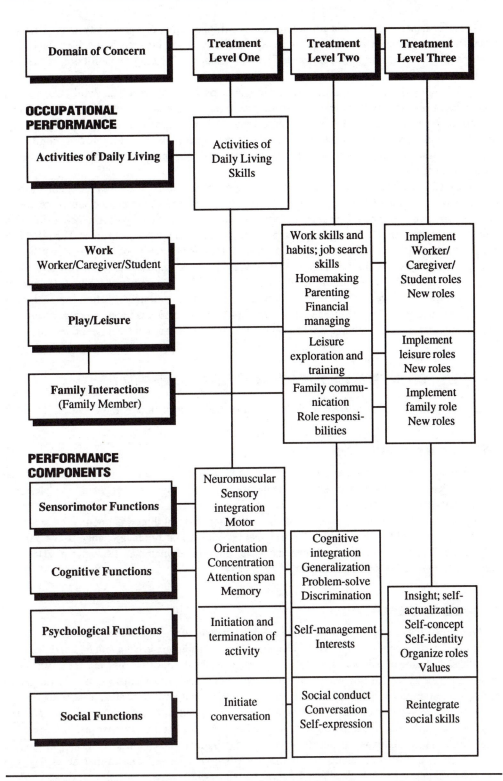

Figure 4-2. Relationship among treatment levels and occupational performance and performance components.

social performance components are addressed at a higher level of complexity than what was appropriate for treatment level one. Psychosocial skills focus on interests and self-management. In terms of social skills, social conduct is fostered through enhancing the ability to express the self.[12]

Activities of daily living skills are no longer a problem at treatment level two, but the occupational therapy performance areas of work (eg. home management, care of others, education, vocation, etc.) and leisure require remediation.[12] Family interaction skills are also developed, but only with regard to enhancing communication skills and improving family role responsibilities. Relapse prevention is another treatment category that receives attention at treatment level two.

Treatment level three focuses on a set of problems different from the treatment emphasis of the other two treatment levels. In order to progress to treatment level three, the substance abuser no longer demonstrates cognitive, social, sensorimotor or occupational performance difficulties. This does not mean that the occupational therapist can afford to ignore these areas. The reliability of the substance abuser's adaptive coping is tenuous. Monitoring or the occasional strengthening of the newly developed skills is required. However, the main emphasis of treatment level three is upon the psychological issues of the addiction, particularly in terms of enhancing self-concept. Self-awareness, self-identity, self-expression and ultimately self-actualization are targeted. Developing a crystallized value set that supports sobriety and decision making is crucial. Organizing performance behaviors into new roles is another important treatment concern.

◆ INTERACTIVE TREATMENT VARIABLES ◆

What treatment variables interact with the identified characteristics of the substance abuser?

TREATMENT VARIABLES

Treatment variables involve the concept of PDS status. PDS status incorporates the three treatment levels that were delineated in response to corresponding changes in the preferred defense structure. At level one, the PDS is mobilized, and at level two, the PDS is weakened. Finally, the PDS is thoroughly confronted by completion of level three treatment.

Treatment variables also include the treatment methods that produce change in the PDS at each level. Directive methods mobilize the PDS, supportive methods weaken the PDS, and confrontational methods prevent continued PDS usage.

FRAMES OF REFERENCE

Obviously, the therapist must be familiar with a variety of frames of reference, since no one frame of reference applies equally to all substance abusers. Addiction is not a unitary condition. Not only does one frame of reference fail to meet the needs of all substance abusers, but using one frame of reference exclusively is not always effective throughout the three treatment levels. Some frames of reference address the particular issue inherent in a treatment level better than others do.

Table 4-2 compares of the frames of reference described in this book as important in the treatment of substance abusers. These frames of reference include: a) management of cognitive disabilities, b) action-consequence (behavioral), c) cognitive-behavioral, d) model of human occupation, and e) object relations. For the reader's convenience, sources that describe these frames of reference in more detail are listed in the appendix.

Table 4-2
Applicability of Frames of Reference to Treatment Levels

Frame of Reference	Treatment Level 1	Treatment Level 2	Treatment Level 3
Action-Consequence	X	X	
Cognitive-Behavioral		X	
Management of Disabilities	X		
Model of Human Occupation	X	X	X
Object Relations			X

According to Table 4-2, two frames of reference, ie. cognitive-behavioral and object relations, are not compatible with treatment level one requirements. The object relations frame of reference prematurely mobilizes the PDS and creates unnecessary confrontation. A cognitive-behavioral approach focuses on internal control when external control is more effective in producing initial abstinence.

Certain frames of reference are not compatible with the treatment level two issue of developing internal control. For treatment level two issues, object relations is not suitable. This frame of reference fails to delineate methods of coping and fails to incorporate a supportive treatment approach. Rather than weaken overreliance on the PDS, the object relations frame of reference strongly confronts any maladaptive defense mechanisms. Also not appropriate for treatment level two is management of cognitive disabilities. This frame of reference maintains too much control with the therapist and does little to develop the substance abuser's internal control. A directive treatment style typical of management of cognitive disabilities is not compatible with the need for a supportive approach.

As was true of the other treatment levels, several frames of reference do not meet the requirements of treatment level three. Because of the need for confrontational treatment methods that promote self-awareness, the management of cognitive disabilities and action-consequence frames of reference are not considered appropriate. Obviously, action-consequence and management of cognitive disabilities frames of reference do little to encourage introspection. These frames of reference emphasize external control of behavior through environmental manipulation and reinforcement. The cognitive-behavioral frame of reference is limited in terms of facilitating the examination of the major issues surrounding drug use. However, a type of self-examination occurs through the cognitive-behavioral approaches of listening to internal "tapes" as a precursor for developing more positive thinking.

Frames of reference must also correspond, when possible, to the therapist involved, facility and setting. These factors usually change due to the fact that the treatment levels integrate inpatient and outpatient therapy over a period of several years. Ultimately, being able to select the most appropriate frame of reference requires skilled clinical reasoning.[2]

◆ OUTCOMES OF TREATMENT MATCHING ◆

What is the anticipated outcome of this interaction between treatment variables and the characteristics of the substance abuser?

OUTCOMES

Outcomes are the expected results of the interaction between characteristics of the substance abuser or PDS variables, treatment variables and the frame of reference. Outcomes are specified for each treatment level and include abstinence at level one, improved coping at level two, and personality development at level three.

OUTCOME MEASUREMENT

Ideally, outcomes are measured as improvements in baseline measurements taken at the beginning of each treatment level. Specific measurement tools used for this process depend upon the frame of reference selected. At the beginning of treatment level one, data identifying loss of control over substance use and overreliance upon the PDS are contrasted to later evidence indicating abstinence and PDS mobilization. In terms of successful mobilization of the PDS, the occupational therapist notes acceptance of addiction as a problem (selective denial), sober rationalizations, acknowledgment of similarities with other substance abusers (assimilative projection), obsession with sobriety, attending to the process of achieving abstinence rather than focusing on other distracting problems (selective attention), etc. Changes in occupational component dysfunction and in ADL performance are compared to pretreatment level one measurements.

Coping deficits, delineated through the evaluation process at the beginning of treatment level two, are contrasted to the improvement in these coping skills once treatment level two is completed. In this way, it is possible to determine whether the substance abuser is ready to progress to treatment level three. Improvements in work and leisure performance and in higher level occupational component skills are noted as well.

At the beginning of treatment level three, level of insight and the state of personality growth are assessed for later comparison once treatment has focused upon these problem areas. Values and interests that support sobriety are assessed as well. Ability to perform in newly developed roles are also evaluated. These measures determine readiness for treatment discontinuation.

◆ TIMING OF MATCHING DECISIONS ◆

When should these matching decisions be made?

SCREENING

After a substance abuser is admitted to an inpatient or outpatient treatment facility, the occupational therapist begins the screening process, which is composed of a chart review, interview or the use of self-report instruments and performance observation.[13, 14] Screening identifies the PDS variables or characteristics of the substance abuser to be addressed in treatment. The PDS variables are synthesized into a tentative list of strengths and weaknesses. Depending on the strengths and weaknesses, a particular treatment level is selected that corresponds to the main therapeutic issue, ie. external control at treatment level one, internal control at treatment level two or insight at treatment level three.

Most substance abusers have problems from each level. The lowest level with a significant number of problems is selected as the major issue for treatment. A frame of reference is then chosen based upon the PDS variables and the PDS status. The frame of reference assists the occupational therapist in more fully understanding the PDS variables. The tentative strengths and weaknesses are further analyzed and formulated through in-depth evaluation once the frame of reference has been selected.

REEVALUATION

As the PDS status improves or regresses, the therapist determines if a change in the frame of reference is required. Because frames of reference address PDS variables in a differential manner, there is a need to constantly assess whether the selected approach is effectively dealing with the PDS variables. According to Mattingly, clinical reasoning enables the therapist to continually respond in a fluid manner to new patient information and a changing treatment environment.[2] Reevaluation ensures that the desired outcome is achieved.

Determining PDS status change is similar to the initial screening process and may use performance testing and observation, interview, or the gathering of data from treatment team members, the medical record or significant others. Only the necessary data-gathering techniques are employed, unlike the screening process that involved a mandatory procedure of chart review, interview and performance observation.

◆ DETAILS OF FRAME OF REFERENCE SELECTION ◆

The initial frame of reference selection process is now outlined in more detail. Measurement tools to assess PDS variables and PDS status changes (level progression and regression) are suggested. To demonstrate the frame of reference selection process, note the manner in which a patient diagnosed with substance dependence is tracked from admission through the screening process. These principles of screening are applicable to both inpatient or outpatient settings. Assume that the occupational therapist received a referral for evaluation and treatment. If the referral is appropriate, the therapist begins the frame of reference selection process.

CHART REVIEW

The first screening step involves a chart review. A chart review form is helpful in organizing chart information so that only pertinent data are selected. In addition to the usual information headings of diagnosis, medications, presenting problems, mental status, precautions and history, the chart review ascertains pertinent PDS variables. PDS variables of the substance abuser indicate need for external control, internal control, or insight.

Table 4-3 lists possible chart data corresponding with a particular PDS variable. Figures 4-3 through 4-5 are sample completed chart review forms, illustrating each corresponding PDS status. It is doubtful that new admissions to an inpatient treatment program would be classified at treatment levels two or three. Note that the chart review sample for level three involved a patient entering an outpatient program after completing inpatient treatment.

INTERVIEW OR SELF-REPORT INSTRUMENTS

An interview follows the chart review. Before the interview proceeds, the occupational therapist ascertains whether the substance abuser is capable of participating in the process. Occasionally, due to medical instability and/or severe cognitive deficits, the interview is delayed until the substance abuser's condition improves. The interview assesses the characteristics of the substance abuser that indicate a particular treatment level.

Table 4-3 is used not only to gather chart information, but also to help organize unstructured interview questions and resulting data. Occupational therapy structured interviews may be used as long as the interview is analyzed in terms of the PDS variables. One interview, The Occupational Case Analysis Interview and Rating Scale, has been partially analyzed as an example and is illustrated in Table 4-4.[15]

Interviews that focus upon only one major PDS variable (Table 4-5) may also be selected. This is especially helpful when trying to differentiate between treatment levels one and two. The therapist may want to limit data gathering to current defense mechanisms used, locus of control or psychological status. Review of the literature revealed a self-report instrument, The Defense

Table 4-3
Chart Data and Corresponding PDS Variables

Characteristics of the Alcoholic

External Control	Internal Control	Emotional Development
Dependency symptoms	Abstinent	Extended period of abstinence
Loss of control	Mobilized PDS	Weakened PDS
Defense mechanisms	Support system	Intact coping skills
a. Denial	Few enablers	Limited insight
b. Rationalization	No depression	a. Self-awareness
c. Projection	Few stressors	b. Self-identity
d. Dichotomous thinking	No cognitive impairment	c. Self-expression
e. Conflict avoidance	No psychosis	d. Self-actualization
f. Selective attention	Limited coping	Lack of crystallized value set
g. Passivity	a. Assertiveness	Need for expanded role behavior
h. Obsessional focusing	b. Stress management	
i. Nonanalytical modes of thinking	c. Problem-solving	
Lack of support system	d. Social skills	
Presence of enablers	Limited role performance	
Depression	Limited insight	
Multiple stressors	Unclear values	
Cognitive impairment		
Psychosis		
Poor habits		
Low self-esteem		
External locus of control		
Poor coping skills		
Role impairment		
Poor insight		
Negative change in values		

Patient Name _____   **Date** ____9/7/93____
Admission Date ____9/6/93_____   **Referral Date** ____9/6/93__
Physician _____   **Treatment Team** ____3__
Referral ____Evaluation and treatment of functional performance deficits____
Diagnosis ____Alcohol dependence_____
Medications ____Librium_____   **Age** ____42_____
Precautions ____Suicidal_____   **Employment** None____

Presenting Problems Pt. has been drinking approximately 2 pints of vodka per day. Pt was divorced from his wife one month ago and lost his job on 8/23/93. Pt. has been feeling increasingly depressed in the last two weeks. Pt. called his eldest son on the evening of 9/6/93 threatening to shoot himself. His son was able to stop him.

History Pt. has been drinking on and off for five years. This is the patient's first treatment for alcoholism. Pt. was married for 15 years and had four children, all males. The eldest son is 20. Pt. lives alone as all his children live with his exwife. Pt. is a lawyer and worked for a prestigious law firm until his dismissal on 8/23/93.

Mental Status Neat appearance; relevant conversation; alert; depressed mood; appropriate affect; anxious (perspiring, moist hands, wringing hands); hesitant thinking; suicidal thought; oriented Xs 3; remote and recent memory intact; short attention span; able to calculate; demonstrates abstract thinking (parable); adequate judgment; lacks insight into problems and relationship to drinking.

PDS Variables (External Control) Dependence syndrome; lack of support system; suicidal; depression; reports multiple unsuccessful attempts to quit drinking; blames others for his problems; ambivalent about the role of drinking in current problems; many stressors including recent divorce, loss of job and financial problems.

PDS Status Level 1

Figure 4-3. Sample chart review form. External control.

Mechanism Inventory, capable of analyzing the substance abuser's defense structure. The Defense Mechanism Inventory has been used in several studies to examine differences between alcoholics and nonalcoholics in terms of defense mechanisms.[16, 17]

In addition to the type of defense mechanisms employed by the substance abuser, the state of the defense mechanisms can be ascertained. The Alcohol Use Inventory examines the substance abuser's level of denial associated with alcohol abuse.[18] The instrument contains 17 scales reflecting perceived benefits of alcohol to the patient, concomitance of alcohol use, disruptive consequences of drinking, patient concerns about the use of alcohol, and the extent to which the patient acknowledges having a drinking problem.

Two other self-report instruments are also useful in ascertaining level of denial and its effect on motivation for treatment. The Assessment of Life Experience Scale (ALE) examines the substance abuser's degree of satisfaction with four dimensions of life, ie. housing accommodation, job satisfaction, financial situation and social life.[19] The Motivation Scale measures the substance abuser's willingness to ameliorate problems of addiction. A sample item asks, "If you

Patient Name		Date	9/7/93
Admission Date	9/6/93	Referral Date	9/6/93
Physician		Treatment Team	3
Referral	Evaluation and treatment of coping skills deficits		
Diagnosis	Alcohol abuse		
Medications	None	Age	42
Precautions	None	Employment	Lawyer

Presenting Problems   Pt. has been abstinent for two weeks. Pt. reports difficulty in managing urges to drink although has resisted temptation thus far. Pt. reported difficulty coping with feelings and sharing problems with family. Pt reports marital problems and very little interaction with his three sons. Pt. also states that his job offers no potential for advancement and has become uninteresting and boring.

History   Prior to the two week period of abstinence, pt. drank on and off for a period of five years. Pt. has never previously received treatment for alcohol abuse.

Mental Status   Neat appearance; relevant conversation; alert; appropriate affect and normal mood; hesitant thinking; oriented Xs 3; remote and recent memory intact; adequate attention span; able to calculate; demonstrates abstract thinking (parable); adequate judgment; insight into problems and relationship to drinking.

PDS Variables   (Internal Control) Abstinent, lacks coping skills, has a shaky support system, admits problems with alcohol, role impairment, and intact cognitive skills.

PDS Status   Level 2

Figure 4-4. Sample chart review form. Internal control.

associate with people who are a bad influence on you as far as drinking is concerned, would you be willing to avoid them?"[19]

An interview can also examine internal versus external locus of control. The first two treatment levels are differentiated by the nature of control necessary to produce adaptive functioning. Level one is characterized by the need for external control, whereas level two consists of a shift to internal control. It must be cautioned, though, that Rotter's Locus of Control Scale (IE) has produced contradictory results with substance abusing populations.[20]

Substance abusers tend to score in a more internally-oriented direction than do those who do not abuse substances.[21, 22] The expectation is for the substance abuser to score like other psychiatric patients in the direction of externality. There may be an optimum internal-control score. The substance abuser's perception of control may be excessively internally-oriented. This would, in fact, be consistent with the need for external control in order to maintain abstinence. External control of the reinforcement provided by alcohol and other drugs may be necessary in order to overcome this excessive and unrealistic belief in one's internal control as effective in countering significant life problems. Abstinence fosters a more realistic appraisal of one's capabilities.

Another important consideration for the interview is the extent of any psychological complications. There is agreement on the prevalence of depressive affect among substance abusers. However, it is difficult to draw conclusions about the clinical relevance of these symptoms. Within

Patient Name _____   **Date** ___9/7/93_____
Admission Date ___9/6/93_____   **Referral Date** ___9/6/93___
Physician: _____   **Treatment Team** ___3_____
Referral ___Evaluation and treatment of personality deficits_____
Diagnosis ___Alcohol abuse_____
Medications ___None_____   **Age** ___42_____
Precautions ___None_____
Employment ___Lawyer_____

Presenting Problems ___Pt. has completed a 28 day inpatient treatment program prior to admission to the outpatient treatment program. Pt. reports a positive family history of alcoholism and that he has not dealt with issues related to childhood experiences with his alcoholic father. Pt. feels unsure of his ability to remain sober but feels that applying coping strategies learned in treatment will help.___

History ___Pt had been drinking for five years prior to treatment. This was his first hospitalization for alcohol abuse. Pt was having marital problems but family was involved in the patient's treatment program. Pt. plans to return to his position with a law firm as a lawyer.___

Mental Status ___Neat appearance; relevant and spontaneous conversation; alert; appropriate affect and normal mood; oriented Xs 3; remote and recent memory intact; adequate attention span; able to calculate; demonstrates abstract thinking (parable); adequate judgment; insight into problems and relationship to drinking; expresses concern regarding influence of father's drinking on current behavior.___

PDS Variables ___(Insight) Unresolved issues related to family history of alcoholism, family support of recovery, and return to steady employment.___

PDS Status ___Level 3_____

Figure 4-5. Sample chart review form. Insight.

four weeks of abstinence, depressive symptoms abate without antidepressant medication or specific therapeutic interventions for depression.[23-25] Apparently, initial levels of depression are not predictive of prolonged depressive symptoms. The caveat is that depression influences the degree of treatment participation and is associated with poorer treatment outcomes.[26-29]

The occupational therapist may find self-report measures of depression, self-esteem or self-concept useful. The measures of depression include the Zung Self-Rating Scale for Depression, the Hamilton Depression Rating Scale and the Beck Depression Inventory.[30-32] As an adjunct to the self-report measures of depression, Zung developed a depression rating scale that is completed by the therapist after the interview.[33] Self-esteem measures, such as the Tennessee Self-Concept Scale, may also be helpful in identifying the need for level one treatment approaches.[34]

PERFORMANCE MEASURES

Both the chart review and the interview serve a dual purpose. These tools gather information about the substance abuser's characteristics, but they also help determine the focus of the performance measure. Amount of time available for screening is usually a factor, so performance observation is typically limited to one structured test or several quick unstructured observations.

For example, if the chart review and the interview point out the possibility of cognitive deficits, the performance measure determines the nature of these cognitive problems and their effect upon independent functioning. Cognitive problems could prevent progression to treatment levels two and three. Level two employs teaching as the treatment method in order to augment the substance abuser's coping strategies. Level three relies on the substance abuser's ability to abstract in order to develop insight. Several cognitive evaluations appropriate for this determination are listed in Table 4-5 along with other types of performance measures to be discussed later.

Table 4–4
Preferred Defense Structure Interview Analysis

Sample Use of the Occupational Case Analysis Interview and Rating Scale (OCAIRS) to Analyze Preferred Defense Structure (PDS) Variables

Model of Human Occupational Components	Sample OCAIRS Questions	Information Indicating PDS Variables
Volitional Subsystem		
Personal causation	What accomplishments, skills, or talents are you most proud of?	Internal control vs external control
Values and goals	What things are most important for you or do you value in your life?	Erosion of values by substance abuse; evidence of guilt
Interests	How do you like to spend your time?	Dominated by substance abuse; restricted interests; limited participation
Habituation Subsystem		
Roles	When people ask you what you do, what do you tell them?	Evidence of role disruption
Habits	Do you generally have a daily schedule that lets you do the things you need to do and want to do?	Organized around substance usage
Performance Subsystem		
Skills	In your daily activities, what things do you know how to do well?	Denial of problems; grandiosity; level of recognition of substance addiction effect on skills
Occupational Components		
Output	Overall, how satisfied are you with how you spend your time?	Denial; rationalization; projection
Physical environment	Are there any activities you do not participate in because you do not have enough money?	Recognition of limitations imposed by substance usage
Social environment	Who are the most important people in your life right now?	Level of external motivation to quit use of substances
Feedback	How do you know when it is time for you to make a change?	Denial; openness to feedback; recognition of effect of substance abuse on others
Historical	What are some examples of when you were doing the best?	Recognition of changes due to progressive substance abuse

Table 4-5
Interview and Performance Measures

Cognitive Evaluations	Defense Mechanism Evaluations	Locus of Control Evaluations	Psychological Evaluations	Occupational Performance Evaluations
Allen Cognitive Level Test (ACL)	Alcohol Use Inventory	Locus of Control-Chance Scale	Beck Depression Inventory	Comprehensive Eval of Basic Living Skills (CEBLS)
Allen Cognitive Level-Problem Solving Version (ACL-PS)	Assessment of Life Experience Scale (ALE)	Rotter's Locus of Control Scale	Hamilton Depression Rating Scale	Kohlman Eval of Living Skills (KELS)
Bay Area Functional Performance Evaluation (BAFPE)	Defense Mechanism Inventory		Tennessee Self Concept Scale	Milwaukee Eval of Daily Living Skills (MEDLS)
Cognitive Adaptive Skills Evaluation (CASE)	Motivation Scale		Zung Self-Rating Scale for Depression	Scorable Self-Care Evaluation (SSCE)
Comprehensive Occupational Task Evaluation Scale (COTE)				
Dynamic Investigation				
Loewenstein OT Cognitive Assessment Battery (LOTCA)				
Luria Nebraska Screening Test				
Mental Status Exam				
Task Skill Observations				

Cognitive Assessment

By understanding the process of detoxification, the therapist embraces the importance of cognitive-oriented screening as the primary focus for the performance measure. Cognitive testing is not always indicated. However, the therapist needs to make absolutely sure that this is really the case. Even those substance abusers who appear high functioning verbally may be masking subtle cognitive deficits. In fact, the ability of 54 male alcoholic inpatients to recall and recognize elements of a film on alcoholism indicated that performance remained significantly impaired two to three weeks after their last drink.[35]

The Bay Area Functional Performance Evaluation (BaFPE) and the Allen Cognitive Level Test provide cognitive functioning data.[36-37] Masagatani, Nielson and Ranslow developed the Cognitive Adaptive Skills Evaluation (CASE), which examines an individual's cognitive process while performing a task (making a calendar).[38] Results are expressed in terms of performance summaries giving the occupational therapist an idea of effect of cognitive deficits upon functioning.

The Loewenstein Occupational Therapy Cognitive Assessment Battery (LOTCA), originally developed for use with brain injured patients, has been studied to determine applicability to psychiatric populations.[39-40] The Luria Nebraska Screening Test is another possibility for determining cognitive problems, especially when the cognitive deficits are subtle.[41] In those cases in which the cognitive deficits are grossly apparent, the Luria Nebraska Screening provides relatively little new information. After committing eight errors on the Luria Nebraska Screening, the test is discontinued as this is an indication of cognitive problems. More specific testing is then conducted in order to gather details of the cognitive problems.

In lieu of a standardized performance measure of cognition, data can be ascertained through an addendum to a general interview and observation of task skills.[42] In the interview, the therapist takes note of particular kinds of behavior, eg. general responsiveness, grooming, manner, speech, mood and emotions. The therapist also asks specific cognitive oriented questions related to orientation, memory, concentration, insight, judgment and problem solving, thought processes, mental content and knowledge. In other words, a mental status type interview can be useful. The interview is followed by observation of task skills. The substance abuser is required to use tools and materials, organize the activity sequentially, follow directions, problem-solve, etc. The Comprehensive Occupational Task Evaluation Scale can be used to record the cognitive observations contributing to task performance.[43]

The previously described cognitive evaluations primarily identify cognitive deficits or deficit task abilities thought to reflect cognitive dysfunction. Occupational therapy evaluations that examine information processing skills and learning potential are currently in various stages of development.[44-46] Toglia refers to the methodology used in examining information processing as dynamic investigation.[44-45] According to Toglia, dynamic investigation involves the gradual introduction of external cues to reveal learning potential, use of cognitive strategies, and responses to different types of feedback or task modifications.[44-45] In other words, increasingly structured cues are provided to facilitate performance. The evaluation task is graded according to test environment, test familiarity, directions, response rate required, etc.

Josman and Katz developed a problem-solving version of the Allen Cognitive Level Test (ACL) that is a type of dynamic investigation.[47, 36] This version uses the same test materials and task as the ACL. In the problem-solving version (ACL-PS), the subject replicates the completed leather lacing stitches without demonstration. Verbal instructions are provided if the subject cannot replicate the stitches. Demonstration is then provided if verbal instructions alone are not conducive to problem solving. In this way, the evaluator assesses problem solving ability dynamically by varying the external cues provided.

Dynamic investigation has an advantage over base-line evaluations. Deficit specific evaluations only indicate substandard performance. Dynamic investigation determines the underlying factors that contribute to the cognitive problem, as well as those factors that facilitate cognitive performance.

For example, consider a substance abuser who demonstrates adequate task skills until attempting to complete an unfamiliar task. Engagement in an unfamiliar task produces difficulty recognizing errors. Problem recognition is enhanced, however, when a repetition cue is given by the therapist that asks the substance abuser to look again to determine whether a mistake was made. Strategy questioning by the therapist regarding the substance abuser's difficulty in noticing task errors, reveals that the substance abuser feels overwhelmed when confronted with novel tasks and has difficulty selectively attending to relevant details. Selective attention is subsequently facilitated when the novel task is presented in a familiar environment and the rate of task performance is slowed.

Defense Mechanism Assessment

Performance measures may also assess the status of defense mechanisms and the role that these defenses play in the substance abuser's interpersonal interactions. Because the state of the substance abuser's preferred defense structure determines readiness for successive treatment levels, it is logical to evaluate overreliance upon certain defense mechanisms. The problem, of course, is to find a performance measure that rates observed defense mechanism utilization.

It is possible to observe the substance abuser's interpersonal interactions and to make subjective assessments regarding use of defense mechanisms. Behavioral examples of denial, projection, rationalization and dichotomous thinking are gathered in terms of interference with the substance abuser's ability to obtain abstinence, to enlist alternative coping strategies and to gain insight.

For example, the substance abuser, when asked to participate in leisure planning, selects activities that previously involved drug consumption, eg. bowling or baseball games. Denial of substance abuse seriously restricts healthy leisure role development. Another example is the substance abuser who consistently avoids assertively expressing needs to the group. Conflict minimization and passivity are the defense mechanisms in operation.

Locus of Control

Actually, locus of control may indirectly measure cognitive impairments and abnormal defense mechanism usage. External locus of control is associated with greater psychopathology, a relationship that holds true for addicted populations.[21, 48] Researchers have reported that external substance abusers tend to be more anxious, depressed, alienated and, in general, more clinically pathological.

In terms of cognitive style, the literature shows that "internal" substance abusers utilize field-independent strategies, while "externals" are more likely to use field-dependent strategies.[49-51] Field-dependent persons are defined as those "who are unable to make accurate perceptual judgments divorced from contextual cues of the field."[52] Field-independent persons are defined as those "who appear to function at relatively higher levels of cognitive articulation and psychological complexity."[52]

As was the case for defense mechanisms, locus of control is subjectively assessed through observation. Relying on others to make decisions, assuming a victim stance by blaming others for problems incurred, or avoiding long-range planning due to reliance on fate are all examples of external locus of control behaviors. Excessive internal control is demonstrated by refusal to seek help when indicated, difficulty adapting to situations beyond one's control, displaying overly perfectionistic behaviors, or consistently taking over leadership roles even when not desirable to do so.

Psychological Assessment

Brown and Schuckit determined that dysphoric mood dominates the depressive symptom pattern of recently detoxified substance abusers.[53] These mood-related symptoms change rapidly over time within a four week detoxification period. Vegetative symptoms commonly associated with depression, however, are the most resistant to change over the first month of abstinence. A history of more severe withdrawal symptoms and more limited social supports are associated with clinically significant levels of prolonged depression.[54-55]

The occupational therapist observes the depressive behavior, carefully noting vegetative symptoms that interfere with functional performance. Vegetative symptoms of depression include sleep disturbances, changes in appetite with resulting weight loss or gain, decreased energy, psychomotor agitation or retardation, difficulty concentrating and loss of interest in sexual activity.

Occupational Performance

Performance observation may need to focus upon self-care abilities involving grooming, oral hygiene, bathing, nutrition, dressing and safety awareness. Several ADL tools are appropriate including the *Milwaukee Evaluation of Daily Living Skills*, the *Kohlman Evaluation of Living Skills*, the *Scorable Self-Care Evaluation*, and the *Comprehensive Evaluation of Basic Living Skills*.[56-59] Unstructured observations of selected self-care tasks are useful as well.

SYNTHESIS AND TREATMENT LEVEL ASSIGNMENT

Table 4-3 is used to synthesize the data from the chart review, interview and performance measure into tentative strengths and weaknesses reflective of a particular treatment level. A frame of reference is selected that capitalizes on the substance abuser's PDS variables.

Screening involves a brief but concerted effort to differentiate the substance abuser's level of functioning. It is probable that most substance abusers require level one treatment at least during the detoxification phase. The therapist should not, however, fall into the trap of automatically utilizing level one treatment approaches for everyone just because they are a new referral. Some substance abuser's detoxify very rapidly. Some may not be physiologically addicted but are abusers of various substances. For these persons, there are no complications related to withdrawal. Also, there are always those cases, for whatever reason, that were not referred to occupational therapy until later in the rehabilitation process. The point is that some substance abusers do not need level one approaches, or if they do, the need is short-lived due to rapid recovery and resulting progression in the PDS status.

◆ CONCLUSIONS ◆

In this chapter, groundwork was provided by describing a method of selecting a frame of reference through the use of screening data. Screening data includes a chart review, an interview and a performance measure. The frame of reference selection process was modified with the three hierarchical treatment levels, corresponding to progressive changes in the substance abuser's preferred defense structure.

Chart review forms that not only gathered the typical background information of the substance abuser, but that also selected pertinent PDS data, were provided. Patient interview methods were selected based on PDS data that could be ascertained. A sample analysis of a standardized occupational therapy interview was partially completed to demonstrate how the information could be interpreted in terms of PDS variables. Performance measures that focused on cognitive performance, defense mechanism utilization, locus of control, psychological state and occupational performance were delineated.

References

1. Rogers J, Holm MB: The therapist's thinking behind functional assessment I. In CB Royeen (Ed.): *AOTA Self Study Series Assessing Function.* Rockville, MD: American Occupational Therapy Association, 1989, pp. 1-32.
2. Mattingly C: Perspectives on clinical reasoning for occupational therapy. In SC Robertson (Ed.): *Mental Health FOCUS Skills for Assessment and Treatment.* Rockville, MD: American Occupational Therapy Association, 1988, pp. 81-88.
3. Gibbs LE: A classification of alcoholics relevant to type-specific treatment. *Int J Addict* 15(4): 461-488, 1980.
4. Annis HM, Chan D: The differential treatment method: Empirical evidence from a personality typology of adult offenders. *Crim Just Beh* 10: 159-173, 1983.

5. Glaser F: Anybody got a match? Treatment research and the matching hypothesis. In G Edwards, M Grant (Eds.): *Alcoholism: Treatment in Transition.* London: Groom Helm, 1980.
6. Glaser FB, Greenberg, SW, Barrett, MA: *A Systems Approach to Alcohol Treatment.* Toronto, Canada: Addiction Research Foundation, 1978.
7. Kissin B, Platz A, Su W: Social and psychological factors in the treatment of chronic alcoholism. *J Psychiatr Res* 8(1): 13-27, 1970.
8. Lyons JP, Welte JN, Brown J, Sokolow L, Hynes G: Variation in alcoholism treatment orientation: Differential impact upon specific subpopulations. *Alcohol: Clin Exper Research* 6: 333-343, 1982.
9. Pattison EM: The selection of treatment modalities for the alcoholic patient. In JH Mendelson, NK Mello (Eds.): *The Diagnosis and Treatment of Alcoholism.* New York: McGraw-Hill Book Co., 1979.
10. Finney JW, Moos RH: Matching patients with treatments: Conceptual and methodological issues. *J Stud Alcohol* 47(2): 122-134, 1986.
11. Moyers PA: An organizational framework for occupational therapy in the treatment of alcoholism. *Occ Th MH* 8(2): 27-46, 1988.
12. American Occupational Therapy Association Uniform Terminology Task Force: Uniform Terminology for Occupational Therapy, 2d ed. *Am J Occup Ther* 43(12): 808-815, 1989.
13. Denton PL: *Psychiatric Occupational Therapy: A Workbook of Practical Skills.* Boston, MA: Little, Brown and Company, 1987.
14. Denton PL, Skinner ST: Selecting a frame of reference/practice model. In Robertson SC (Ed.): *FOCUS Skills for Assessment and Treatment.* Rockville, MD: The American Occupational Therapy Association, Inc., 1988, pp. 100-108.
15. Kaplan K, Kielhofner G: *Occupational Case Analysis Interview and Rating Scale.* Thorofare, NJ: Slack, 1989.
16. Gleser G, Ihilivech D: An objective instrument for measuring defense mechanisms. *J Consult Clin Psychol* 33: 51-60, 1969.
17. Aldridge R, et al: *Defense Mechanisms of an Alcoholic Population as Compared to a Normal Population.* Master's thesis, Michigan State University, 1967.
18. Wanberg KW, Horn JL, Foster FM: A differential assessment model for alcoholism: The scales of the Alcohol Use Inventory. *J Stud Alcohol* 38: 512-543, 1977.
19. Smart R, Gray G: Multiple predictors of dropout from alcoholism treatment. *Arch Gen Psychiatry* 35: 363-367, 1978.
20. Rotter JB: Generalized expectancies for internal vs. external control of reinforcement. *Psychol Monogram* 80 (Whole No. 609): 1-28, 1966.
21. Goss A, Morosko TE: Relation between a dimension of internal-external control and the MMPI with an alcoholic population. *J Consult Clin Psychol* 34: 189-192, 1970.
22. Distefano MK, Pryer MW, Garrison JL: Internal-external control among alcoholics. *J Clin Psychol* 28(1): 36-37, 1972.
23. Hesselbrock M, Babor TF, Hesselbrock V, Meyer RE, Workman K: "Never believe an alcoholic?" On the validity of self-report measures of alcohol dependence and related constructs. *Int J Addict* 18: 593-609, 1983.
24. Jaffe JH, Ciraulo DA: Drugs used in the treatment of alcoholism. In Mendelson JH, Mello NK (Eds.): *The Diagnosis and Treatment of Alcoholism.* New York: McGraw-Hill, 1985, pp. 355-389.
25. Willenbring ML: Measurement of depression in alcoholics. *J Stud Alcohol* 47: 367-372, 1986.
26. Hammen LL, Peters SD: Interpersonal consequences of drinking: Responses to men and women enacting a depressed role. *J Abnorm Psychol* 87: 322-332, 1978.
27. Howes MJ, Hokanson JE: Conversational and social responses to depressive interpersonal behavior. *J Abnorm Psychol* 88: 625-634, 1979.
28. Hatsukami D, Pickens RW: Posttreatment depression in an alcohol and drug abuse population. *Am J Psychiatry* 139: 1563-1566, 1982.
29. Pettinati HM, Sugerman AA, Dibonato N, Maurer HS: Natural history of alcoholism over four years after treatment. *J Stud Alcohol* 43: 210-215, 1982.
30. Zung WK: A self-rating depression scale. *Arch Gen Psychiatry* 12: 63-70, 1965.
31. Hamilton M: Development of a rating scale for primary depressive illness. *Br J Soc Clin Psychol* 6: 278-296, 1967.
32. Beck A, et al: An inventory for measuring depression. *Arch Gen Psychiatry* 4: 53-63, 1961.
33. Zung WK: The depression status inventory: An adjunct to the self-rating depression scale. *J Clin Psychol* 28(4): 539-543, 1972.
34. Fitts WH: *Manual: Tennessee Self-Concept Scale.* Los Angeles, CA: Western Psychological Services, 1965.
35. Becker JT, Jaffe JH: Impaired memory treatment-relevant information in inpatient men alcoholics. *J Stud Alcohol* 45: 339-343, 1984.
36. Allen CK: *Occupational Therapy for Psychiatric Diseases: Measurement and Management of Cognitive Disabilities.* Boston, MA: Little Brown, 1985.

37. Bloomer J, Williams S: The Bay Area Functional Performance Evaluation. In Hemphill B (Ed.): *The Evaluative Process in Psychiatric Occupational Therapy*. Thorofare, NJ: Slack, 1982, pp. 255-308.

38. Masagatani GN, Nielson CS, Ranslow ER: *Cognitive Adaptive Skills Evaluation Manual*. New York: Haworth Press, 1981.

39. Najenson T, et al: An elementary cognitive assessment and treatment of craniocerebrally injured patients. In Edelstein B, Couture E (Ed.): *Behavioral Assessment and Rehabilitation of the Traumatically Brain-damaged*. New York: Plenum Press, 1984.

40. Averbuch S, Katz N: Assessment of perceptual cognitive performance: Comparison of psychiatric and brain injured adult patients. *Occ Th MH* 8(1): 57-71, 1988.

41. Golden C, Hammerse T, Purisch A: *The Luria-Nebraska Neuropsychological Battery*. Los Angeles, CA: Western Psychological Services, 1980.

42. Mosey AC: *Psychosocial Components of Occupational Therapy*. New York: Raven Press, 1986.

43. Brayman SJ, Kirby TF, Misenhamer AM, Short MJ: Comprehensive occupational therapy evaluation scale. *Am J Occup Ther* 30: 94, 1976.

44. Toglia JP: Approaches to cognitive assessment of the brain-injured adult: Traditional methods and dynamic investigation. *Occup Ther Practice* 1(1): 36-57, 1989a.

45. Toglia JP: Visual perception of objects: An approach to assessment and intervention. *Am J Occup Ther* 43(9): 589-595, 1989b.

46. Abreu BC, Toglia JP: Cognitive rehabilitation: A model for occupational therapy. *Am J Occup Ther* 41(7): 439-448, 1987.

47. Josman N, Katz N: A problem-solving version of the Allen Cognitive Level Test. *Am J Occup Ther* 45(4): 331-339, 1991.

48. Harrow M, Ferrante A: Locus of control in psychiatric patients. *J Consult Clin Psychol* 33: 582-589, 1969.

49. Erickson RC, Smyth L, Donovan DH, O'Leary HR: Psychopathology and defensive style of alcoholics as a function of congruence-incongruence between psychological differentiation and locus of control. *Psychol Rep* 39: 51-54, 1976.

50. Donovan DM, Hague WH, O'Leary MR: Perceptual differentiation and defense mechanisms in alcoholics. *J Clin Psychol* 31(2): 356-359, 1975.

51. Ihilevich D, Gleser GC: Relationship of defense mechanisms to field dependence-independence. *J Abnorm Psychol* 77: 296-302, 1971.

52. O'Leary MR, Donovan DM, Kasner KH: Shifts in perceptual differentiation and defense mechanisms in alcoholics. *J Clin Psychol* 31(3): 565-567, 1975.

53. Brown SA, Schuckit MA: Changes in depression among abstinent alcoholics. *J Stud Alcohol* 49(5): 412-417, 1988.

54. Nakamura MM, Overall JE, Hollister LE, Radcliffe E: Factors affecting outcome of depressive symptom in alcoholics. *Alcohol Clin Exp Res* 7: 188-193, 1983.

55. Overall JE, Reilly EL, Kelley JT, Hollister LE: Persistence of depression in detoxified alcoholics. *Alcohol Clin Exp Res* 9: 331-333, 1985.

56. Leonardelli CA: *The Milwaukee Evaluation of Daily Living Skills: Evaluation in Long-Term Psychiatric Care*. Thorofare, NJ: Slack, 1988.

57. Thomson LK: *Kohlman Evaluation of Daily Living Skills (KELS)*. Rockville, MD: AOTA, 1992.

58. Peters M, Clark N: *Scorable Self-Care Evaluation*. Thorofare, NJ: Slack, 1984.

59. Casanova JS, Ferber J: Comprehensive evaluation of basic living skills. *Am J Occup Ther* 30: 101-105, 1976.

Assessment and Treatment
Level One

INTRODUCTION

Once the screening process is complete, treatment level one approaches are dependent to some extent on the frame of reference selected. Not all occupational therapy or psychosocial frames of reference address the major issue of needing external control to achieve abstinence. This chapter identifies several frames of reference important for assisting the substance abuser in obtaining sobriety.

Once the frame of reference has been selected, in-depth evaluation occurs. Evaluation specifies in greater detail the substance abuser's functional strengths and weaknesses as previously identified by the screening process. From the data, an occupational therapy functional diagnosis is formulated as a basis for treatment planning. Treatment goals are specified with corresponding individual strategies and group methods designed to improve occupational functioning. The therapist enlists a directive therapeutic style during treatment level one in order to mobilize the PDS.

◆ FRAMES OF REFERENCE ◆

Frames of reference appropriate for use during treatment level one are those that employ directive approaches and that are capable of addressing the characteristic occupational component and occupational performance problems. Recall from Chapter 4 that ADL issues are typical of treatment level one. The occupational component dysfunction usually involves cognition, particularly orientation, level of arousal, recognition, attention span and memory. Socialization difficulties involve problems interacting with others. Conduct inconsistent with social norms is exhibited. Psychological deficits involve difficulty initiating and terminating activity appropriately. Sensorimotor issues result from impaired neuromuscular, sensory integration and motor functioning.[1]

Several occupational therapy frames of reference are effective for treatment level one. Management of cognitive disabilities, action-consequence and the model of human occupation are three examples of appropriate frames of reference. Figure 5-1 indicates the capability of these three frames of reference in addressing level one treatment problems.

MANAGEMENT OF COGNITIVE DISABILITIES

Management of cognitive disabilities frame of reference examines the relationship between cognitive functioning and sensory cues. Allen describes a voluntary motor action as a "behavioral response to a sensory cue that is guided by the mind."[2] Six cognitive levels represent differential responses to sensory cues at varying levels of consciousness. These responses consist of a continuum of behaviors, ie. automatic, imitated or spontaneous. This frame of reference clearly meets the requirement inherent in level one for providing external control. Attention is given to structuring the external environment for the purpose of maximizing existing cognitive functioning.

The strongest aspect of this frame of reference is its ability to monitor neuropsychological changes during the detoxification process. Therapists determine when the substance abuser is cognitively ready to benefit from treatment that relies on the ability to learn and abstract in order to gain insight. Additionally, because cognitive deficits may affect the substance abuser's ability to participate in traditional verbal treatment, a program can be designed that maximizes participation. Complex activity steps are modified to correspond with the substance abuser's remaining cognitive processing abilities.

ACTION-CONSEQUENCE

The action-consequence frame of reference is appropriate for use during treatment level one due to its emphasis upon reinforcement for the maintenance of behavior. This frame of reference applies behavioral theories in the learning of occupational behavior. The pivotal theoretical assumption is that behavior is predictable, measurable and objective.[3] A person has a repertoire of both adaptive and maladaptive behaviors learned through selective reinforcement from the environment. This behavioral repertoire affects the individual's ability to function in societal roles. A person can learn to modify and control behavior through differential reinforcement and through the systematic application of learning techniques.

In occupational therapy, evaluation determines the extent of maladaptive behaviors and their frequency as associated with substance abuse. The stimuli that cue the substance abuse behaviors are identified in order to either remove these stimuli or desensitize the substance abuser's reactions to them. Existing adaptive and missing behaviors necessary for functioning without the

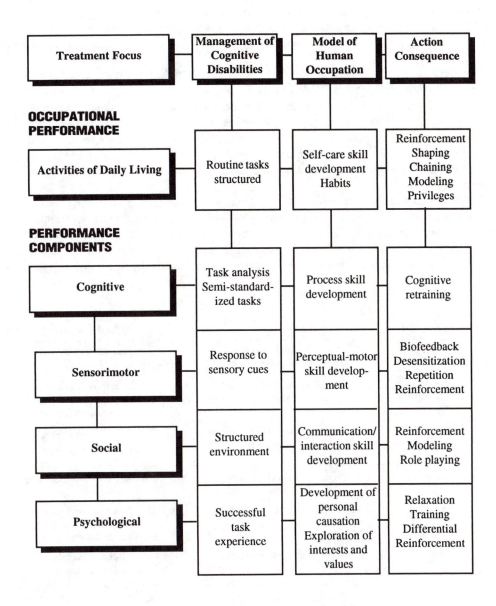

Figure 5-1. Level one treatment focus in three frames of reference. At level one, PDS=Mobilized;   Treatment outcome=Abstinence

use of chemicals are delineated. Reinforcers and the manipulators of reinforcement are analyzed in order to determine the sources of motivation for adaptive, sober behavior.[4] Activities are utilized to teach specific adaptive skills, to provide simulated learning experiences, and to serve as reinforcement.[4] The occupational therapist uses reinforcement to establish new behaviors and eventually to promote the generalization of these new skills to a range of appropriate situations.

MODEL OF HUMAN OCCUPATION

Figure 5-2 indicates the applicability of the model of human occupation. The model of human occupation views people as complex open systems.[5] Due to interaction with the environment, the system is constantly in a state of flux. Information from the environment enters the human system through intake. Information is then processed and integrated into the system via throughput. Once processed, output or occupational behavior results, providing feedback to the system.[5]

The throughput system is composed of three subsystems arranged in hierarchical order. The volitional subsystem governs the system through the choosing and initiating of occupational behavior. The volitional subsystem consists of personal causation, values and interests. The middle level or the habituation subsystem organizes occupational behavior into roles and habits. Production of occupational behavior is relegated to the lowest level or the performance

Subsystems	Function	Effects of Dependency
Volitional	**Choose and Initiate Occupational Behavior**	**Loss of Self-control**
Personal causation	Choose actions	Shifts in locus of control Impaired self-efficacy Expectation of failure
Values	Attribute meaning and set goals	Obsession with substance abuse
Interests	Prioritize activity choices	Centered on substance abuse
Habituation	**Organize Occupational Behavior**	**Substance Abuse Dominated**
Roles	Prescribe use of time and standards for competence	Poor role performance Job and marital difficulties Decreased community involvement
Habits	Organize temporal behaviors	Pathological habits Decreased self-care
Performance	**Produce Occupational Behavior/ Mobilize Skills**	**Loss of Current and Potential Skills**
Communication/interaction skills	Share and receive information and coordinate behavior	Poor social skills
Process skills	Plan, problem-solve and organize action in time and space	Neuropsychological deficits Decreased learning ability
Perceptual motor skills	Interpret input and manipulate self and others	Neuropsychological deficits

Figure 5-2. Application of the model of human occupation to substance abuse.

subsystem. The performance subsystem includes three types of skills involving communication/ interaction, process and perceptual motor abilities.

In terms of the volitional subsystem, substance abuse affects personal causation by creating shifts in locus of control. Both external and excessively internal locus of control have been documented in substance abusers.[5] Values of the substance abuser reflect positive expectations for chemicals to alter mood states. The substance abuser's interests are restricted to those activities in which using is considered acceptable. The habituation subsystem is affected through disruptions in family and work roles. Habits are organized around using routines. Social skill deficits occur when drugs serve as coping mechanisms in times of low self-efficacy. Unfortunately, addiction eventually interferes with the future learning of alternative, more healthy interaction styles. Process and perceptual motor abilities are influenced by the type, amount, frequency and total duration of drugs abused.

◆ OCCUPATIONAL THERAPY DIAGNOSIS ◆

FUNCTIONAL EVALUATION

Once the frame of reference has been selected, the occupational therapist proceeds with the functional evaluation. The evaluation identifies the major functional problems to be addressed during treatment level one. The occupational therapy diagnosis can then be specified, thereby updating the tentative list of strengths and weaknesses previously synthesized from screening data. Problems and strengths are revised according to a clearer picture of the substance abuser obtained by in-depth evaluation.

Table 5-1 lists evaluations by frame of reference that further analyze the treatment level one cognitive, psychological, social, sensorimotor and ADL problems. Evaluation normally begins, however, with the occupational performances creating the most problems in terms of community adjustment. The substance abuser or the family has probably indicated these concerns during the screening interview or chart review.

For example, the wife might state that the substance abuser is extremely forgetful, has trouble getting up in the morning, and is often late or absent from work. The employer might complain that the quality of work has decreased and that problem-solving seems superficial. The memory difficulties, decreased arousal and poor problem-solving suggest that cognitive deficits interfere with occupational functioning. Evaluations are consequently selected that examine underlying cognitive factors and their relationship with occupational performance.

Because cognitive deficits related to substance abuse have been demonstrated in as many as 75 percent of the addicts entering treatment, in-depth cognitive evaluation is often the best starting point for the functional evaluation.[6] Failure to discern the existence of cognitive deficits can lead professionals to conclude that poor performance by substance abusers in treatment results from lack of motivation or lack of desire to quit using. In actuality, cognitive deficits may produce learning difficulties that interfere with participation in an intensive treatment program. Cognitive functioning is a modest predictor of successful substance abuse treatment outcomes.[7-9]

Toglia delineated a variety of approaches for evaluating the cognitive performance of brain-injured adults.[10] Toglia's evaluation classification system is helpful in determining the specific evaluation capable of analyzing the substance abuser's suspected cognitive problems. According to Toglia, cognitive evaluations can be divided into those that delineate functional cognitive performance, determine cognitive levels of functioning, evaluate cognitive deficits, ascertain impaired processing skills, and measure learning potential.[10]

Table 5-1
Treatment Level One Evaluations

Treatment Level Problems

Frame of Reference	Cognitive	Psychological	Social	Sensorimotor	Activities of Daily Living
Cognitive Disabilities	ACL LCL ACL-PS LOTCA	N/A	N/A	N/A	Routine Task Inventory Routine Task History Interview
Action Consequence	BaFPE CASE Elizur QNST ACL ACL-PS LOTCA	State-Trait Anxiety Inventory IPAT Anxiety Scale Questionnaire (Self-Analysis Form)	BaFPE SIS Scale COTE	N/A	CEBLS KELS Scorable Self-Care MEDLS Activity Configuration Barth Time Construction
Model of Human Occupation	BaFPE CASE Elizur QNST ACL ACL-PS LOTCA Dynamic	Internal/External Scale Hopelessness Scale Tennessee Self-Concept Scale Self-Esteem Scale	OCAIRS COTE BaFPE SIS Scale	SBC Person Symbol VMI VOT MSRT MVPT Purdue Peg Board	CEBLS KELS Scorable Self-Care MEDLS OCAIRS Time Reference Inventory Occupational Performance History Interview

Cognitive functional performance evaluations either determine the cognitive deficits (eg. attention, memory, etc.) that interfere with functional task performance or identify the activity components with which the person has difficulty as a result of cognitive deficits. Figure 5-3 gives examples of occupational therapy evaluations that fit into Toglia's classification scheme and that are useful in the evaluation of substance abusers' cognitive performance.

FUNCTIONAL ASSESSMENT

The occupational therapy assessment is differentiated from the functional evaluation process. The purpose of assessment is to synthesize data from records, observations, interviews and standardized testing in order to document the functional status of the individual. The functional status includes the functional diagnosis, the functional change already occurring since admission, and the functional prognosis of the patient.[11]

Recall from Chapter 1 that the functional diagnosis describes the occupational role or

FUNCTIONAL PERFORMANCE

Cognitive Deficits Influencing Performance
Bay Area Functional Performance Evaluation (Bloomer and Williams, 1982)

Cognitive Adaptive Skills (Masagatani, Nielson and Ranslow, 1981)

Difficult Activities
Routine Task Inventory Evaluation (Allen, 1985)

COGNITIVE LEVELS

Allen Cognitive Level Test (ACL) (Allen, 1985)

COGNITIVE DEFICITS

Loewenstein Occupational Therapy Cognitive Assessment (LOTCA) (Itzkovitch, Elazar and Aberbuch, 1990)

IMPAIRED PROCESSING

Dynamic Investigation (Toglia, 1989)

LEARNING POTENTIAL

Allen Cognitive Level Test Problem-Solving Version (Josman and Katz, 1991)

Figure 5-3. Occupational therapy cognitive evaluations based on Toglia's classification. *From Toglia JP: Approaches to cognitive assessment of the brain-injured adult: Traditional methods and dynamic investigation. Occ Ther Practice 1(1):36-57, 1989.*

performance function/dysfunction. The functional diagnosis indicates the medical necessity for occupational therapy intervention. According to Rogers and Holmes, a diagnosis also indicates the underlying performance components that contribute to the role or task performance dysfunction.[12] Specific cues that illustrate component deficits are listed and the relationship to pathology is clearly delineated.

Given the previous example (see Functional Evaluation, above), the occupational therapy diagnosis is derived from the wife's and the employer's reports regarding the role dysfunction and the observation of performance during a typical work task identified as an aspect of the substance abuser's job. Figure 5-4 outlines an occupational therapy diagnosis.

Role Dysfunction	High incidence of absenteeism from work. Quality of work is not meeting expectations of employer. Does not recognize alcohol's impact on role performance (max assist).
Performance Dysfunction	Needs moderate assist (cognitive cuing) in performing routine work tasks, such as preparing financial reports.
Component Dysfunction	Cognitive problems related to decreased arousal, attention span, selective attention, memory loss and problem-solving.
Cues	BaFPE Cognitive score below the mean. Dynamic investigation reveals interruption of task performance related to short attention span and difficulty selectively attending to relevant stimuli. Uses inefficient problem-solving strategies and continues to try the same strategies even though proven ineffective.
Pathology	Alcohol dependence.

Figure 5-4. Occupational therapy level one diagnosis.

When cognitive evaluations are used as the in-depth evaluation measure, certain problems arise. Most cognitive evaluations typically provide details regarding the presence or absence of cognitive component functioning. For example, the cognitive evaluation determines intact or deficit skills in orientation, memory, judgment, etc. There are few clearly defined relationships between cognitive component functioning and independence in occupational functioning. Consequently, determining the functional diagnosis and prognosis of the substance abuser is difficult. To improve the therapist's ability to infer functional performance of the substance abuser from a variety of cognitive evaluation data, cognitive components can be classified into three main categories.[13] Normal task performance depends upon the general cognitive functions of capacity, content and control.

Capacity functions are closely tied to the individual's level of arousal.[13] These functions enable the individual to hold on to information. Capacity functions include attention and short-term memory.[13] Content functions give meaning to objects, physical actions and mental operations.[13] Meaning is generated from perceptual information and from long-term memory. Control functions, mediated through language, regulate behavior by generating and/or inhibiting thoughts and actions. Control functions involve selective attention, implementation of learning strategies (verbal rehearsal or visualization), encoding information to improve recall (chunking), initiating active search to discern relationships between natural categories, compensating for perceptual deficits, and organizing goal-directed activity.[13]

The substance abuser's cognitive assessment data is organized into the three categories of capacity, content and control functions. Predictions regarding task performance can be made by understanding that not all tasks make the same demands upon these three main functions.[13] Low capacity tasks include habitual activities that involve automatic processing of information. Tasks requiring higher capacity are those that involve intentional learning, semantic rather than perceptual processing, time limits, or the holding of information in short-term memory for increasing lengths of time.

In terms of content functions, tasks are made more demanding when the number of meaning dimensions (objects, actions and operations), is increased. Content complexity increases as concrete information becomes more abstract, perceptual differentiation between objects is less obvious, and a larger number of items requires recognition.[13] Nonroutine tasks that require thinking, judging, planning or synthesizing new information place greater demands upon control functions.

The occupational therapy cognitive assessment of the substance abuser includes a description regarding capacity, content and control functions. This information is presented in the cue portion of the occupational therapy diagnosis. Organizing data in this way is more meaningful for treatment planning than simply stating scores on cognitive tests (Figure 5-5).

Functional change indicates the extent of cognitive recovery occurring during detoxification. Particular attention is given to the impact of these functional changes upon task performance. The functional prognosis of the substance abuser is dependent upon the functional change that has occurred since admission and that can be expected to occur given the knowledge of the substance abuser's cognitive deficits. Predictions can be made when comparing the task demands required in the expected environment with the substance abuser's available or potentially available capacity, content and control functions. Figure 5-5 contains a sample cognitive assessment of a substance abuser.

◆ OCCUPATIONAL THERAPY TREATMENT ◆

DIRECTIVE APPROACH

The outcome desired after completing treatment level one is abstinence. In order to achieve abstinence and cope with withdrawal, a directive approach is desired (Figure 5-6). This implements the PDS mobilization process. The therapist deliberately designs strategies that foster assimilative projection and sober rationalizations. A directive style satisfies unmet dependency needs of the substance abuser and ensures that desire for structure is satisfied. Degree of therapy complexity is controlled through directive approaches so that unnecessary cognitive demands are not made upon a detoxing substance abuser. Directive methods also ensure that the substance abuser does not consistently deny drug use as a problem. Manipulative behavior on the part of the substance abuser cannot be tolerated.

A word of caution is necessary at this point. A directive therapeutic style is not to be confused with power struggles.[14] Power struggles are avoided. If a power struggle does occur, this may reflect transference/countertransference issues or may indicate that the PDS is inadvertently being confronted. A period of rapport building is a prerequisite to implementation of a directive style. Being directive also does not mean that principles of empathy, positive regard, respect for human dignity, compassion and honesty are forgotten.[14] Being directive means taking a leadership role with regard to the substance abuser's treatment.

Functional Diagnosis

Role Dysfunction

High incidence of absenteeism from work.
Quality of work is not meeting expectations of employer. Does not recognize alcohol's impact on role performance (max assist).

Performance Dysfunction

Needs moderate assist (cognitive cuing) in performing routine work tasks, such as preparing financial reports.

Component Dysfunction

Cognitive problems related to decreased arousal, attention span, selective attention, memory loss, and problem solving.

Cues

BaFPE Cognitive score below the mean.
Dynamic investigation reveals:

Capacity
Short attention span
Low levels of arousal
Restricted short-term memory

Content
Unable to identify consequences of his actions. Cites vague goals for the future. Reports feeling victimized.

Control
Highly distractible in controlled environments. Difficulty attending selectively to details. Problem-solving not improved with verbal or demonstrated instructions.

Pathology

Alcohol dependence.

Functional Change

(after first 5 days of treatment)

Capacity

Increased attention span from 10 to 15 minutes (structured task, trolled environment)
Improved level of alertness (no difficulty in staying awake during the day)

Content

Identifies simple cause/effect task relationships
Unable to discern cause/effect in social interactions

Control

Screens out mild distractions with minimal assistance
Selectively attends to (familiar) task details
Remembers one-step, demonstrated (novel) task instructions

Functional Prognosis

Requires moderate assist to generalize interpersonal skill training to situations similar to those practiced in the treatment setting. Maximum assist to discriminate between circumstances requiring different interpersonal strategies and to utilize problem-solving in complex situations.

Figure 5-5. Occupational therapy treatment level one assessment.

SUPPORTIVE ATTITUDES

Empathy: Focus on cognitive and psychosocial status

Genuineness: Model "I" messages

Respect: Convey belief in inherent strengths and free will

Self-Disclosure: Model to establish intimate relationship

Warmth: Convey non-verbally and verbally

TOTAL WAY OF BEING

Potency: Demonstrate involvement and enthusiasm

Self-Actualization: Reinforce honesty re: effects of abuse

CHALLENGING STYLE

Immediacy: Focus on reality

Confrontation: Confront denial of addiction; avoid power struggles; watch for transference/countertransference

Concreteness: Deal with specifics in the here and now

Figure 5-6. Treatment level one therapeutic use of self: Directive interactive approach.

TREATMENT PLANNING

In conjunction with the substance abuser, treatment plans are delineated to modify the component or performance dysfunctions identified in the occupational therapy diagnosis. The role of the substance abuser is limited in treatment planning during treatment level one. Using a directive approach, the occupational therapist leads the discussion, watching particularly for denial or employment of other defense mechanisms. Treatment planning may be too confrontational for the substance abuser. In these cases, treatment planning participation is limited to choosing groups and time schedules. Cognitive deficits could also decrease ability to participate in planning with the therapist. However, some participation in treatment planning is always maintained.

Short- and long-term goals are delineated in the treatment plan. Long-term goals are functional goals describing changes in either role or performance dysfunction. The long-term goals extend through treatment level one or the expected duration of detoxification. The long-term goals of treatment level one primarily address ADL functioning or safety issues. Long-term goals are measured in terms of the independence levels or assistance needed in occupational performance after reaching maximum benefit from skilled occupational therapy.[15]

Assistance refers to both the physical and cognitive help required for occupational performance. In terms of cognitive assistance, the assistance levels closely correspond to Allen's cognitive levels.[16] Assistance levels include: Dependent (100 percent assistance or Cognitive Level one); Maximum (75 percent assistance or Cognitive Level two); Moderate (50 percent assistance or Cognitive Level three); Minimum (25 percent assistance or Cognitive Level four); Standby (to prevent errors or Cognitive Level five); and Independence (Cognitive Level six).

Short-term goals more appropriately focus upon the underlying performance components restricting occupational performance. However, even in the short-term goals, the relationship between improvements in the components of functioning and the changes in occupational performance are made clear. For example, the patient will follow demonstrated, one-step task directions with minimum assistance within two days in order to complete the financial reports required for work. The time frame for completion of short-term goals is short and may represent change expected in a single week or even in a couple of days. Figure 5-7 outlines sample goals.

Both the long- and the short-term goals are reasonable expectations for improvement, given the occupational therapy statement of functional change and functional prognosis. For example, it is not reasonable to expect an elderly chronic substance abuser, who does not have a support system and who demonstrates severe cognitive impairments that are not improving with detoxification, to achieve complete independence in ADL functioning.

STRATEGIES

Once treatment goals that correspond to the functional problems are delineated, treatment strategies are identified that represent the skilled application of occupational therapy. Skilled services are those that require the expertise of the occupational therapist.[15] Unnecessarily duplicating the services offered by other professionals and providing therapy that does not require expertise should be avoided. Otherwise, it is not clear why occupational therapy services are medically necessary for the particular substance abuser.

For example, teaching assertiveness is not skilled occupational therapy. However, teaching assertiveness and having the substance abuser apply the skills during a task pertinent for occupational role change is considered skilled.[15] Treatment methods are subsequently described that resolve treatment level one problems related to detoxification, cognitive impairment, sensorimotor deficits, psychological dysfunction, social disruptions and ADL problems.

Detoxification

In terms of detoxification, occupational therapists address the differing symptoms produced during withdrawal. Awareness of the length of withdrawal typical for a given drug, dose and half-life of the drug helps to make decisions regarding readiness for involvement in occupational therapy. The occupational therapist monitors physical complications displayed during participation and is ready to take required precautions. Treatment activities are designed that avoid unnecessary physical demands when the person is subject to a variety of physiological complications. Frequent rest periods or activities of a short duration are appropriate.

Psychological and cognitive complications are monitored and addressed during the initial

Long-Term Goals

1. Pt. will independently reduce unexcused absences from work by 100% (1 month).

2. Pt. will complete simulated work tasks (eg. monthly reports) with standby assistance to point out errors (3 weeks).

Short-Term Goals

1. Pt. will relate influence of drinking upon daily schedule with moderate assistance in order to recognize the relationship between drinking and absenteeism from work (1 week).

2. Pt. will recount with minimum assistance influence of drinking on quality of work performance (2 weeks).

   Method: Occupational Role History, Activity Configuration, Life Styles Group

3. Pt. will successfully complete cognitive task requiring organization, sequencing, and problem solving with minimum assistance (cognitive cuing) for a 20 minute period in order to improve quality of work performance (2 weeks).

   Method: Cognitive Skills Group, simulated work activities

Figure 5-7. Sample treatment level one goals.

---

stages of treatment. Mood disturbances are common for many drug withdrawal syndromes and include depression, hostility, anxiety and irritability. Violence can be a complicating factor, especially when dealing with PCP users. Depending on the drug chronically abused, the individual may display delusional thinking, hallucinations and paranoid ideation. Flashbacks are problematic when treating the LSD abuser.

Sleep disturbances are expected for those who abuse barbiturates and amphetamines. Occupational therapy treats these sleep problems through relaxation and biofeedback techniques and through the use of physical activity to increase energy levels. Long-term use of alcohol necessitates treatment that accommodates cognitive impairment, which would otherwise exclude involvement in typical verbal-oriented treatment programs. Chronic marijuana users often display impairments in motivation. This complication is reflected in the treatment plan.

Cognitive Dysfunction

Because subtle cognitive deficits negatively affect a majority of substance abusers, it is important for treatment to address this occupational component dysfunction.[17, 18] Some cognitive deficits are resolved over time with abstinence.[19, 20] This type of recovery is referred to by Goldman as time dependent.[20] These "time-dependent results of abstinence" progress from marked impairments in cognitive functioning during the early abstinence phase to gradual improvement with the passage of time.[19, 20] Dramatic recovery of cognitive functioning occurs after abstinence (within two to three weeks), and then proceeds slowly thereafter up to one year, depending upon the specific drug abused.[20] Age is apparently an important moderating variable, with younger substance abusers under age 40 showing the greatest recovery.[21] Gender differences in this time and recovery pattern have not been found.[22]

However, recovery of certain cognitive skills is extremely slow, or in some instances, nonexistent.[23] These areas of nonrecovery include visual-spatial abilities, abstract reasoning, nonverbal problem-solving, short-term memory, some types of sensory perception and perceptual-motor integration.[19,24] These persistent cognitive deficits may respond to cognitive remediation.[21,25-29] Improvement in cognitive functioning as the result of carefully selected external stimulation is described by Forsberg and Goldman as experience-dependent recovery.[26]

In occupational therapy, cognitive treatment of substance abusers involves monitoring time-dependent recovery, modifying the treatment environment to the appropriate level of cognitive complexity, teaching compensation strategies for coping with persistent cognitive deficits, and facilitating experience-dependent recovery mechanisms.

Monitoring Time-Dependent Recovery

Allen's cognitive levels assist in monitoring the time-dependent recovery of the substance abuser.[2] The six cognitive levels provide a framework that analyzes the substance abuser's response to the cognitive demands inherent in a given task. The therapist observes the substance abuser's routine task behavior and interprets findings in light of the patient's processing capabilities, the diagnosis (abuse versus dependence), the individual's past experience with the task, and the task's cognitive complexity. Through periodic observation of routine task behavior, the substance abuser's task limitations (cognitive disability) and remaining task abilities become evident.

To determine whether the substance abuser is beginning to perform at the next higher cognitive level, an expectant treatment approach is utilized. According to Allen, "Expectant treatment aims at documenting the alterations and improvements in functional abilities associated with biologic changes in the patient's condition."[2] Expectant treatment requires that the task demand be slightly higher than the current performance. This strategy determines if the substance abuser can produce the task behavior reflective of cognitive improvement.

Modifying the Treatment Environment

Cognitive deficits affect the substance abuser's treatment participation. Reducing the cognitive complexity involves modifying the treatment environment to accommodate the substance abuser's available capacity, content and control functions. Through activity analysis, the occupational therapist determines the cognitive demands made by a task in a given context and matches those demands with the cognitive capabilities of the substance abuser. Allen's cognitive levels are useful in guiding the activity analysis for those substance abusers functioning at cognitive level five or lower.[2] Activities are modified by controlling the processing complexity of the sensory cues inherent within the task.

Modifying the environment to accommodate cognitive limitations is an important aspect of what Allen refers to as supportive and palliative treatment strategies.[2] Supportive treatment, as used within management of cognitive disabilities, is not to be confused with supportive approaches described in this book as necessary for treatment level two. Supportive treatment, according to Allen, "aims at sustaining the patient's strength and is especially important when the patient states that he or she feels hopeless."[2] Supportive treatment illustrates to the substance abuser the remaining cognitive skills that can be capitalized upon.

Supportive treatment is also important in helping the substance abuser connect effect of drug use with cognitive functioning. As neuropsychological changes occur, the therapist points out to the substance abuser the obvious differences in task performance. In this way, denial of addiction as a problem is confronted without unnecessarily confronting other problems the substance abuser is not yet ready to face. Sober rationalization is also encouraged by demonstrating that one needs to be abstinent in order to improve ability to think.

The purpose of palliative treatment is to reduce the "pain and distress associated with symptoms."[2] Facing cognitive limitations is distressful and too much discomfort leads to reliance upon maladaptive defenses, including the abuse of substances. It is certain that a pleasant task experience does more to promote trust and a sense of belonging than does a stressful situation produced due to a mismatch of cognitive demand with functioning level. The structure provided through environmental modification reassures the substance abuser's dependency needs and the desire for predictability.

Teaching Compensation Strategies

Another approach to coping with slow recovering or permanent cognitive deficits, is to teach the substance abuser to compensate for functional impairments. Encouraging the substance abuser to employ compensation strategies for cognitive deficits gives control back to the substance abuser. Dynamic investigation provides the best clues regarding the compensation necessary for facilitating cognitive skill performance. For example, dynamic investigation may reveal that the substance abuser's problem- solving improves when working in a familiar setting, slowing the pace and reducing emotional interference.

The cognitive rehabilitation literature for traumatic brain injury is replete with cognitive compensation strategies that offset memory and problem-solving deficits.[30-31] These techniques may be applicable to substance abusers, depending upon the nature and extent of the cognitive deficits. Some examples of memory compensation techniques include the memory notebook, visual imagery, word association, rehearsal and PQRST (Preview, Question, Reorganize, Self-recite and Test).[30]

Stimulating Recovery

External stimulation may facilitate recovery of persistent cognitive deficits. Research needs to further substantiate these claims. However, positive results have occurred when using visual-spatial practice techniques, hierarchical learning intervention to enhance abstract reasoning, memory training, and concrete or simplified problem-solving training.[21,26-29,32-34]

Improvements in the substance abuser's visual-spatial cognitive functioning result from structured and unstructured practice on visual-spatial tasks, or from practice on task components of the visual-spatial task.[21, 27, 35] Enhanced visual-spatial functioning seems to transfer to other visual-spatial tasks.[26]

Kleinman and Stalcup designed a craft program for a child psychiatric population for the purpose of improving visual-motor skill functioning.[36] The visual-motor skills of the experimental group that engaged in the graded craft program did improve, while controls who participated in a variety of occupational therapy groups did not exhibit the same improvement. Due to the popularity of crafts in substance abuse programs and the visual-motor improvements experimentally facilitated in substance abusers, using crafts with adults to improve visual-motor skills requires investigation.

Improved cognitive processing resulting from practice on visual-spatial tasks designed in the occupational therapy clinic may generalize to other areas of occupational functioning. In fact, Stensrud and Lushbough reported that substance abusers involved in an arts and crafts program significantly improved in the areas of general, interpersonal and task behaviors as measured by the Comprehensive Occupational Therapy Evaluation.[37,38]

Hierarchical learning intervention has been used to modify substance abusers' sorting behavior.[29, 39] These sorting tasks can either require putting objects together or discovering why objects put together belong together. Sorting, a control function, is a measure of abstracting ability, concept formation used in classification, and conceptual flexibility or shifting behavior.[29] Recall that substance abusers demonstrate deficits in all these areas.[40]

According to hierarchical learning intervention, substance abusers are initially trained to organize objects into separate categories according to color.[29] Shifting to the next classification dimension involving form requires the removal of the color dimension. In this way, organization by color is no longer possible and sorting by form becomes immediately obvious. Similarly, shifting to the next classification scheme involving number requires removal of the form dimension.

Once sorting by one dimension and shifting to another single dimension is facilitated, the substance abuser is presented with sorting stimuli containing all three dimensions of color, form and number. Even though all sorting dimensions are present, the substance abuser is required to sort first by color, then to shift sorting using the form dimension, and finally to shift sorting using the number dimension. Signals to shift sorting to another dimension are subtly provided by the therapist who indicates when sorting is correct or incorrect. Of course, the therapist provides demonstration and strategy hints as needed.

Improvement in the memory of substance abusers has resulted from the same memory strategies described previously as methods for teaching compensation, eg. visual imagery, word association, rehearsal, chunking and "PQRST." Whether improvement in memory is resultant from compensation or from actual changes in the brain's memory structures remains to be determined.

In terms of enhancing problem-solving, Wetzig and Hardin taught substance abusers general problem-solving steps at a simplified level of complexity.[29] More advanced problem-solving is addressed during treatment level two. At treatment level one, the substance abusers are helped to solve problems that are already broken down by the therapist into the most simplified form. For instance, a substance abuser might be experiencing difficulty concentrating during the step one meeting (the first stage of the 12-step AA process). Because difficulty concentrating is a complicated problem, the therapist helps the substance abuser redefine the problem more specifically. For instance, "I lose concentration during step one group after about five minutes when other group members are reading out loud the results of their assigned homework to the rest of the group."

With the aid of the therapist, short-term goals that delineate the desired results are set. For example, "I would like to increase my attention to ten minutes so that I can at least hear one group member's completed work." The substance abuser is then assisted in planning strategies that lead to problem solution. The substance abuser lists possible strategies and receives ideas from other substance abusers as well. Ideas for the sample problem might include repeating to oneself essential details of the group member's homework, taking notes or asking others to give feedback when loss of attention is obvious.

Learning from mistakes during problem-solving occurs through the creation of an atmosphere tolerant of experimentation. The substance abuser is aided in recognizing mistakes made during the implementation of problem-solving strategies by the therapist who guides the patient in comparing performance with preset standards. In this way, the substance abuser is taught to make use of feedback in reorganizing problem-solving strategies. For instance, the substance abuser in the previous example records length of time attention is maintained during the group presentations as a method of noting progress over a specified period. If progress is not occurring, the substance abuser is helped to reanalyze the problem, set more reasonable goals or select alternative strategies.

Emphasis in problem-solving is therefore placed on utilizing a systematic "win-stay" approach and avoiding impulsive "lose-shift" styles of problem-solving.[29] In other words, the substance abuser learns that persistence and rational approaches to problem-solving are more effective than impulsively changing strategies at the first sign of mistakes.

Sensorimotor Dysfunction

Treatment of sensorimotor problems related to sensory processing was discussed previously when describing cognitive treatment strategies. Theoretically, sensory perception and cognition are difficult to separate as perception involves such cognitive processes as attention and memory.[41] Sensorimotor skills also involve gross motor abilities, strength and endurance.[1] Biomechanical principles for improving strength and endurance are incorporated into gross motor exercise programs. It is necessary to establish physical exercise as a normal routine.

Frankel and Murphy, through pre- and post-testing of substance abusers, indicated that as physical fitness improved, MMPI scores reflected less psychopathology.[42] Palmer, Vacc and Epstein showed that alcoholics who completed a walking or jogging program three days per week demonstrated significant differences from nonparticipants on measures of state anxiety, trait anxiety and depression.[43] Sinyor, Brown, Rostant and Serganian found that at follow-up abstinence rates were significantly higher for exercisers.[44]

A significant sensorimotor problem affecting chronic alcoholics involves peripheral neuropathies.[45] With the advent of a peripheral neuropathy, the alcoholic experiences problems associated with lack of sensation, decreased muscle strength and decreased fine motor coordination. Depending upon the amount of alcohol routinely consumed and the number of years drinking has ensued, problems associated with the peripheral neuropathy may lessen with detoxification and with vitamin replacement.[45]

However, these problems are unlikely to completely resolve with detoxification. Because peripheral neuropathies are for the most part irreversible, occupational therapy treatment involves compensation. The substance abuser is taught to recognize the safety problems associated with decreased sensation. Fine motor and strength limitations are dealt with through task modifications, learning specialized techniques and adaptive equipment. In terms of task modification, the fine motor demands of a task may be eliminated or completed by others. Using a different lifting strategy to lift heavy items is an example of a specialized technique. Adaptive grips for pencils and pens are examples of the adaptive equipment needed.

Psychological Dysfunction

The psychological dysfunctions typical of treatment level one involve detoxification effects related to anxiety, and depression. Treatment strategies that may lead to a reduction in anxiety involve biofeedback and relaxation training. Depression could be controlled through differential reinforcement of adaptive behaviors. Other psychological problems involve changing the valuing of drugs to the valuing of sobriety. Interests revolving around the use of drugs are replaced with interests that produce the satisfaction that was previously attributed to drug effects.

Detoxification Effects

Anxiety impedes abstinence. Drugs typically have been used to control anxiety.[46] Ability to relax on cue is essential for competing with the powerful relief available from drugs. Biofeedback is effective in reducing anxiety.[47] For best results from biofeedback training, Adler and Adler implement training before complete withdrawal from a particular drug.[47] Relaxation training given during detoxification helps the substance abuser avoid the dysphoria of withdrawal. Excessive frustration with withdrawal dysphoria often contributes to dropping out of therapy.

Earlier, it was learned that depression is one of the main symptoms of detoxification that usually clears once abstinence is maintained. Depression does impede involvement in the treatment program, occasionally leading to early treatment discontinuation. Behaviors exemplifying depression are often expressed as refusal to get out of bed, not eating, lethargy, withdrawn social behavior, tearfulness, hostility, etc. The behavioral methods used to combat the depressive behaviors involve manipulation of differential reinforcement. In other words, a class of adaptive behaviors that is incompatible with the depressive behaviors is reinforced. For example, the substance abuser is required to be up and dressed at a certain time, eat three meals per day, engage in group activity, and employ physical activity to combat lethargy.

Experiencing success is another important factor at treatment level one. Achieving abstinence is the main success along with conquering the ill effects of detoxification. Biofeedback, as discussed previously, is important for enhancing personal causation during detoxification, a time when the substance abuser is most likely to feel "out of control."[47] The substance abuser is encouraged to participate in enjoyable activities in which the pressure to perform according to high standards is minimized. Unconditional acceptance permeates the occupational therapy group climate, fostering assimilative projection.

Values and Interests

Radically changing the value structure of the substance abuser at this treatment level is not appropriate. There are two main value issues that are operating during treatment level one. The value issues revolve around denial and rationalization. Using the principles of selective denial, the substance abuser's valuing of drugs is challenged and replaced with valuing sobriety. Previous values, such as those related to work, family and other social role performances, are capitalized upon in order to develop sober rationalizations. Because the substance abuser wants to succeed on the job and with the family, drug usage is identified as the culprit interfering with desired life outcomes.

If drugs were a major part of the substance abuser's life, past interests were forgotten. Drugs became the most important interest. Interest in sobriety is fostered during treatment level one. This means that sobriety must offer the positive effect previously attributed to drug use. Slavson stated that "activity groups" are important for discovering that the world is not necessarily frustrating, denying and punitive.[48] Previous interests are identified or the substance abuser explores new interests. The substance abuser discriminates between those activities that are especially satisfying and those that either produce little satisfaction or are not enjoyable. Appropriate initiation and termination of activity is an important treatment focus as well.

Social Dysfunction

Social skills are consistently lacking in substance abusers.[49] At treatment level one, social skills are not aggressively developed. In keeping with the concept of mobilizing the PDS, trust in the form of assimilative projection is the main emphasis of socialization at treatment level one. Activities that encourage cooperation are preferred over those that engender competition. The socialization provided within the treatment milieu is important for ensuring that assimilative projection occurs. The substance abuser is taught to trust other recovering substance abusers as persons knowledgable of the suffering characteristic of addiction.

Social skills treatment also considers the social appropriateness of habits.[5] Obviously, drug habits are socially unacceptable and this intolerance for addiction is strongly communicated. The substance abuser is encouraged to examine past drug habits and the resulting influence upon development of social problems. In this way, the substance abuser learns to draw his or her own conclusion that drug habits must be replaced by more satisfying daily routines.

Activities of Daily Living Dysfunction

The occupational therapist is concerned with increasing independence in activities of daily living. Often self-care behaviors of the substance abuser were gravely impaired due to the overinvolvement with obtaining and using the chemical substance. As a result, nutrition, grooming and hygiene were ignored. ADL problems primarily relate to issues of habituation, unless there are complications related to cognitive impairment. Treatment, then, is a matter of reinforcing past successful self-care routines. Direct intervention for activities of daily living is thus reserved for those substance abusers with permanent cognitive deficits, those with underlying pathology such as schizophrenia, or those with social marginality, as is the case for "skid row" alcoholics.

◆ OCCUPATIONAL THERAPY GROUPS ◆

Groups address the performance components and activities of daily living skill deficits exhibited at treatment level one. Groups deliberately mobilize the PDS by encouraging assimilative projection, sober rationalizations and selective denial. Treatment level one groups accommodate PDS issues by delineating expected behavior, reducing conflict, refocusing obsessional thinking, channeling excess energy and capturing attention. The therapist is the group leader, which is consistent with the directive approach concept. Groups at this treatment level are structured and concrete. These group characteristics satisfy the substance abuser's need for external control and management of detoxification.

There are three occupational therapy group types that meet the requirements outlined above. These three group types include milieu therapy, developmental groups and thematic groups. Not all of the developmental groups are appropriate (Table 5-2). Only parallel groups and project groups fit the treatment level one criteria. Thematic groups are defined by Mosey as a "group that focuses on gaining knowledge, skill, and attitudes necessary for mastery of performance components and occupational performances."[50]

MILIEU THERAPY

Milieu therapy is not a treatment in and of itself, but is an "ecological matrix, a metatreatment within which specific treatments can be presented most effectively."[51] Milieu therapy deliberately manages an entire social system in order to maximize therapeutic impact.[52] The nature of the milieu is capable of differentiating highly successful substance abuse treatment programs from less successful ones.[53]

The milieu is an important avenue for mobilizing the PDS. The socialization provided within the treatment milieu facilitates assimilative projection. Feelings of trust are actively promoted through deliberate use of the milieu. For example, planning and implementing Saturday picnics for patients and staff is an activity that promotes closeness between all those participating. The milieu also confronts denial of drug use. Other substance abusers in the treatment program often recognize denial in someone else and confront that individual in an effective manner. The culture of the treatment program transmits "rationalized" beliefs regarding sobriety. The milieu integrates sobriety throughout a normal day, thus refocusing obsessional thinking to sobriety and its corresponding lifestyle. The milieu provides structure that satisfies the need for clear-cut choices and reduction in chaos.

The treatment milieu is an adjunct to traditional occupational therapy groups. The occupational therapist utilizes the milieu as an extension of therapy outside of the formal treatment setting. In this sense, the milieu is utilized by all treatment levels and is not restricted in effectiveness to treatment level one. Practicing new skills, reporting the results of this practice, and observing the behavior of others who possess the desired skills are examples of assignments given to the substance abuser in order to access the potential learning available in the milieu. Knowledge of the PDS mobilization process provides a basis for designing and incorporating milieu structures in substance abuse treatment programs. Occupational therapists could be leaders in milieu design.

Table 5-2
Treatment Level One Groups

Group	Factors to be Considered with Substance Abusers	Strategies
Parallel Group	Ability to work and play in presence of others Cognitive abilities	Unstructured exercise Work activities Individual craft projects
Project Group	Ability for shared interaction and cooperation	Meal preparation Leisure planning Group craft projects
Thematic Group	Level one skill needs of the treatment population	Lifestyle analysis Relaxation ADL

PARALLEL GROUPS

Parallel groups are often associated with craft groups. Within a parallel group, the substance abuser is expected to work at a task in the presence of other group members.[50] Craft groups are important for providing the substance abuser with tasks demanding improvements in memory, organization, attention, concentration, sequencing, planning and problem-solving. In addition to these cognitive skills, crafts can also enhance sensorimotor functioning.

Parallel groups are important for substance abusers experiencing severe interpersonal skills deficits. Parallel groups provide opportunities for developing initial communication skills.[54-57] Incorporating a sharing component into the parallel group design is advantageous.[57] Requiring moderate amounts of sharing seems to increase task engagement over what occurs without any sharing or with too much sharing.[57] The sharing component is important in the process of assimilative projection.

Parallel groups accommodate varying amounts of therapist imposed structure, thus satisfying the substance abuser's dependency needs. Gradual improvements in task performance, as the result of detoxification, are pointed out to the substance abuser. This awareness of cognitive improvement connects effects of past drug use with the previously impaired cognitive performance. This connection challenges denial of drug use as a problem. Parallel groups also channel excess energy into tasks that release aggressive energy in a socially acceptable manner. Time is structured through the use of parallel groups so that drug-related experiences are less likely to be recalled, as might be the case when the patient is bored. Self-esteem is fostered clearly through successful group participation and completion of tasks.

PROJECT GROUPS

The therapist is the leader and takes responsibility for selecting appropriate activities and satisfying group members' needs.[50] In this way, requirements for PDS mobilization are met. The project group differs from the parallel group in that there is an increased demand for interacting with several persons simultaneously. The substance abuser learns how to work with others on a short-term task. The group facilitates assimilative projection by developing relationships through a shared task. Competition is deemphasized. Some examples of appropriate project group tasks include preparing a meal, planning outings, making holiday decorations, planning evening or weekend events, etc.

Other disciplines have described the success of project groups with substance abusers initially seeking sobriety. Holser discussed the failure of a "stress intensity group program" developed for substance abusers coerced into treatment by the legal system.[58] The purpose of the group was to reduce defenses and motivate clients. Holser reported that by the end of the group program, the substance abusers "clung rigidly to their defenses."[58] However, the substance abusers were reluctant to end their participation in the motivation aspect of the group program, consisting of table games, cards, conversation, cooking, serving refreshments, outings and other adult social events.

These conclusions reinforce the concept of mobilizing the PDS prior to confrontation of the maladaptive defense structure. Perhaps, the substance abusers in this program "clung" to their defenses because there were no alternative methods of coping available to them. They enjoyed the trust and mutual support that resulted from social activities conducted within a project group format.

THEMATIC GROUPS

Thematic groups address the specific performance components and/or occupational performance deficits commonly exhibited at treatment level one. Groups remediate cognitive, sensorimotor, psychological, socialization difficulties and ADL deficits. A substance abuser with moderate to severe cognitive deficits benefits from the Directive Group, designed by Kaplan in response to the treatment needs of "acutely ill, minimally functioning patients."[59] The Directive Group incorporates methods of structuring the environment to enhance full participation by all group members.[59]

A thematic group might require the substance abuser to analyze the amount of time devoted to drug use. The group then encourages problem-solving regarding the way in which time can be redirected to sober activity. Emphasis upon reestablishing normal routines and habits are aspects of PDS mobilization properly included in this type of thematic group.

In addition, a thematic group may examine social role performance as it existed while using drugs. The purpose of the group is to mobilize the substance abuser's denial system and to promote sober rationalizations. This is accomplished by having the substance abuser identify the sociocultural problems he or she currently experiences, eg. poor job performance, school failure or difficulty socializing. This highlights the role drug use played in aggravating these problems. In this way, the substance abuser rationalizes reasons for staying sober.

Even though role performance may be impaired as the result of problems other than drug use, these are not dealt with initially. The process of selective denial allows the substance abuser to believe for a limited time that the problems result from drugs. The substance abuser, however, is never allowed to blame his or her drug use on the various problems experienced during role performance. The therapist's function in this group is to assist problem-solving concerning only those issues related to drug use. Problems as a result of immature emotional development are not dealt with at this point in treatment.

Another thematic group might develop strategies for controlling the complications of withdrawal, such as anxiety, depression and restlessness. This group teaches relaxation techniques such as biofeedback, progressive relaxation and physical conditioning. Use of meditation or visual imagery is also helpful. The therapist may need to augment visual imagery techniques with additional structure depending upon the substance abuser's level of cognitive and psychological functioning.

There are many thematic group possibilities that can be designed at treatment level one. The group's focus ultimately depends upon the general needs of the treatment population. For instance, a grooming group may be necessary for "skid-row" alcoholics, but may be unnecessary for middle income substance abusers. The content of the thematic group also depends upon the frame of reference utilized. There may be a specific skill that is not addressed by other treatment groups provided within the milieu that the occupational therapy group can effectively develop strategies to augment. Avoiding unnecessary duplication of services allows the occupational therapist to fill the treatment gaps in the current substance abuse program.

Thematic groups conducted at level one, however, run the risk of assuming characteristics of other treatment level groups before the substance abuser is ready for this progression. This should be avoided unless the group is meant to progress along with the group members' therapeutic progress. This, in fact, may be easier than switching substance abusers from a lower level thematic group to another higher level thematic group. In other words, group members stay in the same group throughout the inpatient stay or the outpatient program. As the group members progress from one treatment level to another, the group changes to reflect the differing PDS status. Until it is clear that treatment level one characteristics are no longer needed, thematic groups retain the necessary PDS characteristics of being structured, concrete and therapist directed.

◆ REEVALUATION ◆

Throughout treatment level one, the occupational therapist continually monitors progress towards the long- and short-term goals. Informal as well as formal data collection strategies are useful. Pre- and post-testing with the same measures used in evaluation are preferred when possible. Completion of the long- term goals signals readiness for treatment level two.

Illustrating medical necessity of the occupational therapy service requires documentation of progress toward treatment level one goals. Lack of progress indicates necessity in making changes in the therapeutic approach, revising the treatment plan to include more realistic objectives, training family members to maintain current levels of progress, or discharging the substance abuser from occupational therapy until status indicates improved readiness for service.

◆ CONCLUSIONS ◆

Treatment level one intervention begins with frame of reference selection. Three occupational therapy frames of reference were appropriate for mobilizing the PDS through the use of directive approaches. Management of cognitive disabilities, action-consequence and model of human occupation were briefly described. Frame of reference selection was followed by functional evaluation, which forms the basis of the occupational therapy diagnosis. Evaluation identifies the underlying cognitive deficits that contribute to role and occupational performance dysfunction.

Assessment involves organizing cognitive data in terms of the substance abuser's capacity, content and control abilities and disabilities. The occupational therapy diagnosis identifies occupational role, occupational performance and occupational component dysfunction and function that can be attributed to addiction. In addition to the diagnosis, the functional status of the substance abuser includes functional changes that have occurred since admission and the functional prognosis.

Treatment planning and reevaluation demonstrate medical necessity. Long- and short-term goals are formulated with the substance abuser's participation. Long-term goals address occupational role or occupational performance dysfunction. Consistent with the functional prognosis, reasonable expectations regarding the assistance levels needed for independent functioning are included. Short-term goals identify achievable improvements in the performance components that restrict occupational performance. Reevaluation monitors progress towards the goals so that changes in the treatment plan are instituted and readiness for treatment level two is determined.

Treatment approaches were described for resolving cognitive, sensorimotor, psychological, social and ADL dysfunctions. Treatment of cognitive dysfunction involved monitoring time-dependent recovery, modifying environments to the appropriate level of cognitive complexity, teaching compensation strategies, and facilitating experience-dependent recovery mechanisms.

Treatment level one groups mobilize the PDS, provide directive approaches and meet the substance abuser's need for external control. Milieu therapy, parallel groups, project groups and thematic groups are enlisted. Parallel groups structured with moderate amounts of sharing are important for task engagement and improving communication skills. Project groups promote communication among group members.

References

1. American Occupational Therapy Association Uniform Terminology Task Force: Uniform Terminology for Occupational Therapy, 2d ed. *Am J Occup Ther* 43(12): 808-815, 1989.
2. Allen CK: *Occupational Therapy for Psychiatric Diseases. Measurement and Management of Cognitive Disabilities.* Boston, MA: Little Brown, 1985, pp. 6, 22, 23.
3. Mosey AC: *Three Frames of Reference for Mental Health.* Thorofare, NJ: Slack, 1970.
4. Bruce MA, Borg B: *Frames of Reference in Psychosocial Occupational Therapy.* Thorofare, NJ: Slack, 1987.
5. Kielhofner G (Ed): *A Model of Human Occupation: Theory and Application.* Baltimore, MD: Williams and Wilkins, 1985.
6. Butters N, Cermak L: *Alcoholic Korsakoff's Syndrome: An Information Processing Approach to Amnesia.* New York: Academic Press, 1980.
7. Abbott MW, Gregson RM: Cognitive dysfunction in the prediction of relapse in alcoholics. *J Stud Alcohol* 42: 230-243, 1981.
8. Guthrie A, Elliott WA: The nature and reversibility of cerebral impairment in alcoholism: Treatment implication. *J Stud Alcohol* 41: 147-155, 1980.
9. Walker RD, Donovan DM, Kivlahan DR, O'Leary MR: Length of stay, neuropsychological performance, and aftercare: Influences on alcohol treatment outcome. *J Consult Clin Psychol* 51(6): 900-911, 1983.
10. Toglia JP: Approaches to cognitive assessment of the brain-injured adult: Traditional methods and dynamic investigation. *Occup Ther Practice* 1(1): 36-57, 1989.
11. Smith R: Synthesizing and interpreting functional assessment data for meaningful recommendations. In Royeen CB (Ed.): *AOTA Self-Study Series: Assessing Function.* (no. 7). Rockville, MD: American Occupational Therapy Association, 1989, pp. 1-36.
12. Rogers J, Holm MB: The therapist's thinking behind functional assessment I. In CB Royeen (Ed.): *AOTA Self Study Series Assessing Function.* Rockville, MD: American Occupational Therapy Association, 1989, pp. 1-32.
13. Vezzetti D: Capacity, content, control: A model for analyzing the cognitive demands of activity. *Occup Ther Practice* 1(1): 9-17, 1989.
14. Small JS: *Becoming Naturally Therapeutic.* Austin, TX: The Eupsychian Press, 1981.
15. Health Care Financing Administration: *Medicare Outpatient Physical Therapy and Comprehensive Outpatient Rehabilitation Facility Manual.* Washington, DC: Author, Transmittal No. 87: 98-111a, 1989.

16. AOTA: *Insuring Payment Through Documentation: A Common Sense Approach.* Workshop held in Washington, DC: 1989, May.

17. Wilkinson DA, Carlen PL: Neuropsychological and neurological assessment of alcoholism. Discrimination between groups of alcoholics. *J Stud Alcohol* 41: 129-139, 1980.

18. Parsons OA, Farr SP: The neuropsychology of alcohol and drug use. In Filskov S & Boll T (Eds.): *Handbook of Clinical Neuropsychology.* New York: Wiley, 1981, pp. 320-365.

19. Goldman MS: Cognitive impairment in chronic alcoholics: Some cause for optimism. *Am Psychol* 10: 1045-1054, 1983.

20. Goldman MS: Neuropsychological recovery in alcoholics: Endogenous and exogenous processes. Alcohol. *Clin Exper Res* 10: 136-144, 1986.

21. Stringer AY, Goldman MS: Experience-dependent recovery of block design performance in male alcoholics: Strategy training versus unstructured practice. *J Stud Alcohol, 49(5): 406-411, 1988.*

22. Silberstein JA, Parsons OA: Neuropsychological impairment in female alcoholics: Replication and extension. *J Abnorm Psychol* 90(2): 179-182, 1981.

23. Brandt J, Butters N, Ryan C, Bayog R: Cognitive loss and recovery in long-term alcohol abusers. *Arch Gen Psychiatry* 40: 435-442, 1983.

24. Hochla NA, Fabian MS, Parsons OA: Brain-age quotients in recently detoxified alcoholic, recovered alcoholic and nonalcoholic women. *J Clin Psychol* 38(1): 207-212, 1982.

25. Forsberg LK, Goldman MS: Experience-dependent recovery of visuospatial functioning in older alcoholic persons. *J Abnorm Psychol* 94: 519-529, 1985.

26. Forsberg LK, Goldman MS: Experience-dependent recovery of cognitive deficits in alcoholics: Extended transfer of training. *J Abnorm Psychol* 96(4): 345-353, 1987.

27. Goldman RS, Goldman MS: Experience-dependent cognitive recovery in alcoholics: A task component strategy. *J Stud Alcohol* 49(2): 142-148, 1988.

28. Yohman JR, Schaeffer KW, Parsons OA: Cognitive training in alcoholic men. *J Consult Clin Psych* 56(1): 67-72, 1988.

29. Wetzig DL, Hardin SI: Neurocognitive deficits of alcoholism: An intervention. *J Clin Psychol* 46(2): 219-229, 1990.

30. Dougherty PM, Radomski MV: *The cognitive rehabilitation workbook.* Rockville, MD: Aspen Publishers, 1987.

31. Carter LT, Caruso J, Languirand MA: *The Thinking Skills Workbook.* Springfield, IL: Charles C Thomas, 1984.

32. Hansen L: Treatment of reduced intellectual functioning in alcoholics. *J Stud Alcohol* 41: 156-158, 1980.

33. Binder JT, Schreiber J: Visual imagery and verbal mediation as memory aids in recovering alcoholics. *J Nerv Ment Dis* 171: 617-623, 1980.

34. Chaney EF, O'Leary MR, Marlatt GA: Skill training with alcoholics. *J Consul Clin Psych* 46: 1092-1104, 1978.

35. Goldman MS: Cognitive impairment in chronic alcoholics: Some cause for optimism. *Am Psychol* 10: 1045-1054, 1983.

36. Kleinman BL, Stalcup A: The effect of graded craft activities on visuomotor integration in an inpatient child psychiatry population. *Am J Occup Ther* 45(4): 324-330, 1991.

37. Stensrud MK, Lushbough RS: The implementation of an occupational therapy program in an alcohol and drug dependency treatment center. *Occup Ther MH* 8(2): 1-15, 1988.

38. Brayman SJ, Kirby TF, Misenheimer AM, Short MJ: Comprehensive occupational therapy evaluation scale. *Am J Occup Ther* 30: 94, 1976.

39. Sanders JA, Sterns HL, Smith M, Sanders RE: Modification of concept identification performance in older adults. *Dev Psych* 11: 824-829, 1975.

40. McCrady BS, Smith DE: Implications of cognitive impairment for the treatment of alcoholism. *Alcohol: Clin Exper Res* 10(2): 145-149, 1986.

41. Trexler L: Cognitive and neuropsychological aspects of affective change following traumatic brain injury. In Trexler L (Ed.): *Cognitive rehabilitation conceptualization and intervention.* New York: Plenum, 1982, pp. 173-197.

42. Frankel A, Murphy J: Physical fitness and personality in alcoholism: Canonical analysis of measures before and after treatment. *Q J Stud Alcohol* 35: 1271-1278, 1974.

43. Palmer J, Vacc N, Epstein J: Adult inpatient alcoholics: Physical exercise as a treatment intervention. *J Stud Alcohol* 49(5): 418-421, 1988.

44. Sinyor D, Brown T, Rostant L, Serganian P: The role of physical program in the treatment of alcoholism. *J Stud Alcohol* 43: 380-386, 1982.

45. Kissin B: Theory and practice in the treatment of alcoholism. In Kissin B & Begleiter H (Eds.): *The Biology of Alcoholism.* Treatment and Rehabilitation of the Chronic Alcoholic, vol. 5. New York: Plenum Press, 1977, pp. 1-51.

46. Kaplan HI, Sadock BJ: *Synopsis of psychiatry, behavioral sciences, clinical psychiatry,* 5th ed. Baltimore, MD: Williams & Wilkins, 1988.

47. Adler CS, Adler SM: Strategies in general Psychiatry. In Basmajian JV (Ed): *Biofeedback Principles and Practice for Clinicians* (3rd ed.). Baltimore, MD: Williams & Wilkins, 1989, pp. 233-248.
48. Slavson S: Group therapy special section meeting. *Am J Orthopsychiatry* 13: 648-690, 1943.
49. Kalin R: Self-descriptions of college problem drinkers. In McClelland DC, et al (Eds.): *The Drinking Man*. New York: Free Press, 1972, pp. 217-231.
50. Mosey AC: *Psychosocial Components of Occupational Therapy*. New York: Raven Press, 1986, p. 289.
51. Abroms G: Defining milieu therapy. *Arch Gen Psychiatry* 21: 553-560, 1969.
52. Pattison E, Coe R, Doerr H: Population variation among alcoholism treatment facilities. *Int J Addict* 8: 199-229, 1973.
53. Costello R: Alcoholism treatment and evaluation: In search of methods. *Int J Addict* 10: 251-275, 1975.
54. DeCarlo JJ, Mann WC: The effectiveness of verbal versus activity groups in improving self-perceptions of interpersonal communication skills. *Am J Occup Ther* 39(1): 20-27, 1985.
55. Schwartzberg S, Howe M, McDermott A: A comparison of three treatment group formats for facilitating social interaction. *Occup Ther MH* 8(2): 1-16, 1982.
56. McDermott AA: The effect of three group formats on group interaction patterns. *Occup Ther MH* 69-89, 1988.
57. Steffan JA, Nelson DL: The effects of tool scarcity on group climate and affective meaning within the context of a stenciling activity. *Am J Occup Ther* 41: 449-453, 1987.
58. Holser MA: A socialization program for chronic alcoholics. *Int J Addict* 14(5): 657-674, 1979.
59. Kaplan K: *Directive Group Therapy Innovative Mental Health Treatment*. Thorofare, NJ: Slack, 1988, p. 22.

Assessment
and Treatment
Level Two

INTRODUCTION

This chapter suggests possible frames of reference that weaken the PDS through teaching alternative coping strategies. The action-consequence, cognitive-behavioral and model of human occupation frames of reference are capable of improving coping and providing supportive treatment approaches.

The occupational therapy diagnostic procedure is described as it relates to treatment level two. Treatment planning is similar to treatment level one, but includes coping skills training and the promotion of internal control. The types of coping skills taught depend upon the drug of choice and the typical response to stress. Relapse prevention is emphasized. Group methods meeting the criteria for treatment level two are identified along with specific reevaluation procedures that determine readiness for treatment level three.

◆ FRAMES OF REFERENCE ◆

A frame of reference is chosen that addresses level two problems, employs a supportive therapeutic style, enhances internal control and develops coping strategies that effectively weaken overreliance on defense mechanisms. The frame of reference meeting these qualifications is more likely to produce improved coping (Figure 6-1). With advancement to treatment level two, most of the cognitive and sensorimotor deficits have been resolved. Higher level cognitive dysfunction at this level involves generalization, discrimination and more complex problem solving skills. Psychosocial skills focus on self-management capabilities and the use of interests as a coping mechanism. Improved social conduct and effective self-expression are the social skills emphasized.[1]

Occupational performance and role dysfunction addressed at treatment level two involve work and leisure. Home management, care of others, education and vocation are defined by Uniform Terminology as work roles.[1] Relapse prevention is also a treatment focus.

ACTION-CONSEQUENCE

The action-consequence frame of reference is appropriate for treatment level two intervention for two main reasons. Contrary to many beliefs, a behavioral approach is useful not only in the development of skills, but also in the enhancement of self-control.[2] This frame of reference focuses on advanced skill training and the engendering of self-control.

Developing self-control is accomplished with the verbal pairing of potential consequences with possible behaviors.[2] Responsibility for the reinforcement of adaptive behavior is turned over to the substance abuser. Teaching coping strategies influences the substance abuser's ability to handle situations that could trigger relapse. In addition, transfer of training techniques contribute to the maintenance of sobriety by ensuring that skills learned during treatment are actually used independently in the home environment.

COGNITIVE-BEHAVIORAL

The cognitive-behavioral frame of reference incorporates some of the more useful components of behaviorism and combines them with cognitive developmental theory. In this frame of reference, cognitions and emotions interact to influence behavior.[3] Both cognitive and behavioral coping strategies are taught that develop the substance abuser's internal control.

Specific cognitive restructuring techniques include challenging faulty thinking, covert problem-solving, stress inoculation and critical incidents.[4] (Many of these techniques are discussed in more detail later in this chapter.) Assertiveness and communications behavioral training are modified to include specific cognitive strategies. Relapse prevention includes teaching cognitive coping strategies, challenging positive expectations of substance use, and strengthening belief in ability to implement new skills successfully.

MODEL OF HUMAN OCCUPATION

The treatment strategies characteristic of the model of human occupation treatment strategies increase the likelihood that the substance abuser will enter into an adaptive cycle of occupational behavior. Adaptive occupational behavior involves engagement in a "balanced routine of work, play and daily living tasks appropriate for their environments, their disabilities and their developmental levels."[5] Occupational dysfunction is the problem focus, and deficits in the

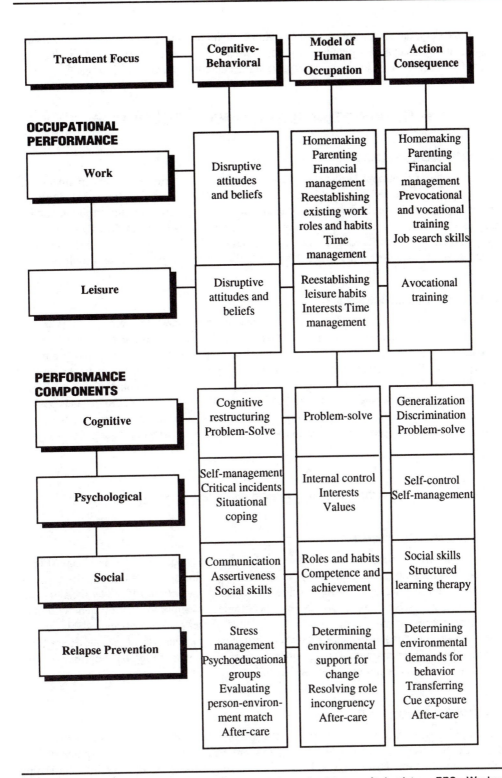

Treatment Focus	Cognitive-Behavioral	Model of Human Occupation	Action Consequence
OCCUPATIONAL PERFORMANCE			
Work	Disruptive attitudes and beliefs	Homemaking Parenting Financial management Reestablishing existing work roles and habits Time management	Homemaking Parenting Financial management Prevocational and vocational training Job search skills
Leisure	Disruptive attitudes and beliefs	Reestablishing leisure habits Interests Time management	Avocational training
PERFORMANCE COMPONENTS			
Cognitive	Cognitive restructuring Problem-Solve	Problem-solve	Generalization Discrimination Problem-solve
Psychological	Self-management Critical incidents Situational coping	Internal control Interests Values	Self-control Self-management
Social	Communication Assertiveness Social skills	Roles and habits Competence and achievement	Social skills Structured learning therapy
Relapse Prevention	Stress management Psychoeducational groups Evaluating person-environ-ment match After-care	Determining environmental support for change Resolving role incongruency After-care	Determining environmental demands for behavior Transferring Cue exposure After-care

Figure 6-1. Level two treatment focus in three frames of reference. At level two, PDS= Weakened; Treatment outcome= Coping.

performance components are interpreted in light of the impact upon occupational performance. Engagement in occupations required by the substance abuser's environment is the main treatment strategy in order to produce adaptive skills and competence in skill usage.[6]

◆ OCCUPATIONAL THERAPY DIAGNOSIS ◆

FUNCTIONAL EVALUATION

As was true of treatment level one, functional evaluation determines the occupational roles and performances affected by component dysfunctions. Evaluation determines the substance abuser's coping skills applied within occupational roles, eg. assertiveness, problem-solving, anger management, etc. Some appropriate evaluation tools include: 1) COPE Inventory of Coping Skills, 2) Gambrill-Richey Assertion Inventory, 3) Problem Situation Inventory, 4) Problem-solving Inventory, and 5) Rotter's I-E Locus of Control Scale (Table 6-1).[7-11]

FUNCTIONAL ASSESSMENT

As was true of treatment level one, the assessment synthesizes the evaluation data into an occupational therapy diagnosis. Figure 6-2 offers an example of a common treatment level two diagnosis. The other components of the functional status are also delineated in the treatment level two assessment. The functional change summarizes progress made as a result of treatment level one intervention. Once treatment level two strategies have been implemented, the functional prognosis predicts improvements in coping and changes in locus of control. Prognosis is positive when evaluation indicates less severe coping and locus of control deficits. A strong support system also improves prognosis. Figure 6-2 also outlines a sample treatment level two assessment.

◆ OCCUPATIONAL THERAPY TREATMENT ◆

SUPPORTIVE APPROACH

Treatment level two requires a different therapeutic style than treatment level one (Figure 6-3). The substance abuser is now ready to assume responsibility for treatment. The therapist employs a supportive manner instead of a directive style of interaction. Efforts by the substance abuser to change behavior are supported by encouraging attempts to develop healthy coping skills. Assertiveness is promoted when the substance abuser makes treatment decisions. Of course, this does not mean that the substance abuser can do whatever he or she desires. The substance abuser functions within the guidelines of the therapeutic program. Program structure is still maintained, but is characterized by flexibility.

TREATMENT PLANNING

Level two treatment planning is similar to the planning process of treatment level one. Long- and short-term goals are delineated in the treatment plan according to the requirements of medical necessity. Long-term goals address either role or performance dysfunctions, indicating the level of assistance that can be achieved by the completion of treatment level two. Short-term

Table 6-1

Treatment Level Two Evaluations

Treatment Level Problems

Frame of Reference	Cognitive	Psychological	Social	Work	Leisure	Homemaking/ Parenting	Relapse
Action Consequence	Problem Solving Inventory	Hassles & Uplifts Scales Ways of Coping Questionnaire COPE Inventory Internal/External Scale Coping Resources Inventory COPE	Social Reticence Scale Gambrill-Richey Assertion Inventory IBS Social Skills Inventory ISI	Independent Living Behavior Checklist KELS Scorable Self-Care Work Behavior Checklist Vocational Skills Evaluation	KELS Scorable Self-Care Interest Checklist Leisure Activities Blank	CEBLS Independent Living Behavior Checklist KELS Scorable Self-Care Independent Living Skills Evaluation	Coping Resources Inventory Problem Situation Inventory Environmental Questionnaire
Cognitive Behavior	Problem Solving Inventory Automatic Thoughts Questionnaire	Hassles & Uplifts Scales Ways of Coping Questionnaire COPE Inventory Internal/External Scale Coping Resources Inventory COPE	Social Reticence Scale Gambrill-Richey Assertion Inventory IBS, VSSI Social Skills Inventory Social Climate Scales ISI	Rahim Organizational Conflict Inventories	N/A	N/A	Coping Resources Inventory Problem Situation Inventory
Model of Human Occupation	Problem Solving Inventory	Internal/External Scale Occupational Questionnaire	Role Checklist Salience Inventory AOF Occupational History Adolescent Role Assessment Role Activity Performance Scale	Independent Living Behavior Checklist KELS Scorable Self-Care Work Behavior Checklist Vocational Skills Evaluation	Interest Checklist Leisure Activities Blank Leisure Satisfaction Scale KELS Scorable Self-Care	CEBLS Independent Living Behavior Checklist KELS Scorable Self-Care Independent Living Skills Evaluation	Pleasant Events Schedule Environmental Questionnaire

Functional Diagnosis

Role Dysfunction	Maximal assist to identify roles that give satisfaction. Views work as overly stressful. Has not received yearly raises due to poor yearly performance evaluations.
Performance Dysfunction	Moderate assist required to cope with aggressive and rude coworkers. Has difficulty completing work tasks on time without standby assist from supervisor.
Component Dysfunction	External locus of control, and lacks stress management and assertiveness skills. Minimal assist to identify stressors on the job.
Cues	Using drugs to cope with conflict and anxiety. Low scores on the Gambill-Richey Assertion Inventory and an external orientation on the Rotter's I-E Locus of Control Scale.
Pathology	Valium and barbiturate abuse
Functional Change	(after completion of treatment level 1)
	No longer denies substance abuse, able to recount impact of using habits upon daily routine, successfully managed detoxification with biofeedback strategies, cognitive deficits have been resolved as noted by improved concentration and recognition of errors, demonstrates trust of other patients and staff.
Functional Prognosis	Support from family members, resolution of cognitive deficits, successfully using a stress management technique to control detoxification, past history of socialization and work performance suggest ability to reach treatment level 2 goals stated in the treatment plan.

Figure 6-2. Occupational therapy treatment level two assessment.

goals address the components restricting performance or role functioning. Figure 6-4 outlines sample treatment level two goals.

The main difference in treatment planning at this level is the role of the substance abuser. The substance abuser directs treatment planning by specifying and prioritizing coping skills, selecting treatment methods and implementing strategies as planned. Planning helps the substance abuser achieve goals that bring emotional satisfaction and eliminate sources of frustration.

STRATEGIES

Coping Issues and Drugs of Choice

As discussed in Chapter 2, coping style is reflected by the substance abuser's drug of choice. These coping styles are activation, relaxation and escape. CNS stimulants are used by those who handle stress through increased arousal. CNS depressants and opioids are methods of obtaining relaxation and withdrawal from stress. Hallucinogens are taken as a method of escape.

SUPPORTIVE ATTITUDES

Empathy: Focus on coping successes

Genuineness: Facilitate non-phoniness

Respect: Allow independent decision-making
and reinforce assertiveness

Self-disclosure: Support
efforts

Warmth: Model and
reinforce

TOTAL WAY OF BEING

Potency: Support enthusiasm
for sobriety

Self-Actualization: Facilitate
"sober" peak experiences

CHALLENGING STYLE

Immediacy: Praise coping efforts

Confrontation: Confront behaviors
compromising internal control

Concreteness: Decode into direct
messages

Figure 6-3. Treatment level two therapeutic use of self: Supportive interactive approach.

Treatment helps the addict achieve these desired states through socially appropriate means. For example, those substance abusers desiring withdrawal from stress are taught relaxation and stress management techniques as substitutes for drug use. Substance abusers using drugs to produce arousal have to substitute daily activities, such as running and other physical exercise, that promote a natural "high". Reducing stress alleviates the uncontrollable need for activation. Specific treatment strategies resolve the need to escape from stress though a drug-induced fantasy life. The occupational therapist examines ways in which a fantasy life can be developed without drugs and can be managed in a socially acceptable way. Writing stories and poetry, acting in plays, or painting are helpful alternatives for those with interests and talent in the creative arts. Escape also is addressed through stress management techniques. Removing oneself from a stressful environment (eg. going on a picnic, taking a walk in the woods or going to a movie) for a period of time promotes physical and psychological renewal. Problems are reframed so that the substance abuser can cope with and solve the dilemma. Perhaps the problem, if reexamined, is not the catastrophe that originally was expected. Alternatives to problem solution that make impulsive escaping unnecessary are beneficial.

Long-Term Goals

1. Pt. will independently complete work tasks on time (3 weeks).
2. Pt. will independently resolve conflicts with coworkers (3 weeks).

Short-Term Goals

1. Pt. will with standby assist identify aspects of work that create stress and prevent timely task completion (1 week).
2. Pt. will with standby assist implement methods to reduce work stress in order to complete work tasks on time (2 weeks).
3. Pt. will independently implement methods to reduce work stress in order to complete work tasks on time (2 weeks).
4. Pt. will assertively express feelings with minimum assistance to rude coworkers (1 week).
5. Pt. will assertively express feelings with standby assist to rude coworkers (2 weeks).

Methods: Stress Management and Assertiveness Training Groups

Figure 6-4. Sample treatment level two goals.

Cognitive Dysfunction

Basic cognitive skill deficits have been resolved prior to advancement to treatment level two. Complex cognitive skills, such as generalization, discrimination and problem-solving, are taught. The substance abuser learns more advanced problem-solving principles and generalizes these skills to apply them to many situations. The substance abuser also challenges specific irrational cognitions that perpetuate abuse of chemicals and other self-destructive behaviors.

Generalization

Generalization is required for learning. Generalization involves a conditioned response being transferred from one stimulus to another.[12] Generalization enhances ability to independently utilize coping strategies taught during treatment level two. Generalization does not occur automatically and therefore must be addressed throughout the treatment level two process. According to Toglia, six basic factors are critical to the generalization process.[13] These six factors include environmental context, nature of the task, learning criteria, metacognition, processing strategies and learner characteristics.

The environmental context refers to the familiarity and the type of environment (eg. crowded, noisy and unfamiliar).[14] The nature of the task involves the demands incurred by the number, material aspects and arrangement of objects requiring manipulation; the task directions; and the physical responses such as postural adjustments and movement patterns.[14] Learning criteria are the standards applied during task performance in order to determine whether learning has actually occurred.[13] Metacognition involves knowledge of one's own cognitive processes as well as monitoring one's own cognitive performance. Processing strategies are used by learners in response to a task. These strategies include selecting relevant information, rehearsing, associating, etc. Learner characteristics involve the learner's previous knowledge, existing skills, attitudes, emotions and experiences.[13]

Generalization is therefore enhanced when the skill being learned is practiced in multiple environments with subtle variations in the task.[13] Variations in the task might include gradually increasing the number of objects to be manipulated or grading the type of directions provided. Progressively more difficult learning criteria, such as a gradual decrease in the number of errors tolerated in performance, are applied to evaluate improvements in learning.[13]

Metacognitive training strategies are taught along with other processing strategies. Examples of metacognitive training strategies include self-estimation, role reversal, self-questioning and self-evaluation.[13] Self-estimation occurs when the substance abuser predicts task difficulty, time to complete the task, errors likely to result and amount of assistance needed. Role reversal is often used in role playing. During role reversal, the substance abuser observes and analyzes the performance of others in order to point out the skill errors. Self-questioning involves stopping periodically in the midst of the task to assess progress. Once the task is completed, the substance abuser assesses through self-evaluation the success of the task performance.[13]

Processing strategies include training in mental rehearsal, visual imagery and other memory enhancement techniques. Planning ahead, prioritizing and removing barriers to performance are other processing strategies.[13] Finally, generalization is facilitated when new learning is deliberately related to previously learned information. Relationships to past learning enhance the meaning of the newly learned skill.[13]

Discrimination

There are specific instances when generalization of learned behaviors is not appropriate. In many circumstances, the ability to discriminate differences between two stimulus events is required to produce the most appropriate behavioral response. Higher learning is dependent upon the balance between generalization and discrimination. Disorders in thinking are often attributable to difficulties with these two cognitive processes. For instance, a recovering alcoholic may generalize that all social events serve alcohol and in order to avoid temptation, decides to restrict all future socialization activities. This example represents both faulty discrimination and generalization.

Discrimination is a part of coping skills training. The substance abuser learns which strategy is the most successful under specific circumstances. Applying the incorrect strategy leads to the faulty conclusion that coping methods are ineffective compared to drugs and maladaptive defense mechanisms.

An important aspect of discrimination is differentiating between sober and addictive behaviors.[15] Wallace describes three discrimination strategies including writing a behavioral inventory of drug use, cognitive behavioral sharpening and naming the addicted person.[15]

Writing a behavioral inventory involves recalling a using episode, writing down the exact circumstances and actions taken and listing the overt consequences. Motivations for drug use are not addressed and there is no attempt to discern reasons for using drugs. The behavioral inventory is then contrasted with the sober responses to similar stimulus events and the resulting differences in experienced consequences.

Cognitive behavioral sharpening is a technique borrowed from Gestalt group therapy.[15,16] The substance abuser is given the choice of two chairs to sit in that are placed in the middle of a group. After being seated, the substance abuser indicates which role will be played, ie. the sober individual or the substance-abusing individual. The substance abuser is then asked to converse with the hypothetical person in the other chair. If the group member has chosen the substance abuser, an interaction with the sober aspect of the self occurs. The exercise develops an identity separation between addictive behaviors and sober behaviors.

Another discrimination method involves naming the substance abusing person.[15] The name reflects self-perception when using drugs. Group members are then divided into pairs in order to discover each other's addictive persona and the meanings behind the names selected.[15]

Differences between behaviors typical when sober and those reflective of using drugs are emphasized.

Problem-Solving

The behavioral skills necessary for problem-solving consist of defining the problem, brainstorming solutions, selecting alternatives, planning implementation steps, implementing the plan, and evaluating effectiveness of the plan.[2, 17] In addition to the behavioral methods, covert problem-solving is taught.

Covert problem-solving begins with cognitive reappraisal.[18] Cognitive reappraisal discriminates among observation, inference and evaluation. The substance abuser reappraises the evaluation that is placed on stimuli. Individuals often confuse evaluation with observation. Observation is closely followed by the process of interpreting factual components of the observation. Typically, not enough data is available. Information gaps are supplemented with inferences that allow one to draw conclusions. Cognitive reappraisal examines possible erroneous evaluations that were based on faulty inferences. Gathering more data helps to decrease reliance on inference so that accurate interpretations ensue.

Pressure or tension generated by inaccurate appraisal is removed when evaluating the stimuli correctly. Relief in pressure gives the substance abuser time to experiment with alternatives to coping with problems by covertly practicing the selected behavioral strategy. Experimentation with alternatives occurs covertly by imagining potential outcomes. The substance abuser then visualizes completing the chosen behaviors successfully.

Irrational Beliefs

Rational-emotive therapy advocates challenging cognitions related to irrational beliefs.[19] Emotional suffering can be attributed to the irrational ways people construe the world. These irrational assumptions lead to a self-defeating internal dialogue that contributes to maladaptive behaviors. In fact, substance abusers have underlying assumptions based on "myths" regarding alcohol.[20] Myths are used to justify drinking, eg. "I drink because of the stress I am currently under."

The substance abuser determines precipitating external events that lead to strong negative emotions. For example, a substance abuser who states he feels angry is encouraged by the occupational therapist to identify a triggering event. Perhaps the substance abuser just received a phone call from his wife indicating that she is unable to attend the AA meeting with him as scheduled. Then, the occupational therapist helps the substance abuser determine the specific thought patterns and underlying beliefs that constitute the internal response to these events. The substance abuser in this example is covertly stating that people should always behave the way he would like them to or that events should go as planned. Next, the occupational therapist helps the substance abuser alter these covert beliefs. The occupational therapist suggests that the substance abuser reformulate this belief so that it is more rational, eg. "Circumstances do not always go as planned and even though I am disappointed, my wife can attend the next evening's AA meeting." Evidence of the substance abuser's thinking style is gathered through activity lists that describe activating events, emotional reactions and corresponding behavioral responses. The substance abuser analyzes the list of the week's activities to put the events into more rational contexts. Analysis of the events creates awareness of assigning peculiar and upsetting meanings to experiences. The substance abuser's "life themes" become evident.[3]

Life themes are the rules for living. Themes might emerge similar to: "Everything bad always happens to me," " No one likes me," or "I am stupid." Corresponding behaviors indicate a pattern of self-destructiveness, dependency or social isolation. Destructive themes and behavioral patterns are indications for cognitive restructuring. Alternative interpretations of these events are offered by the therapist. The substance abuser is taught to independently recognize, monitor and change cognitions produced during routine occupational performances.[21]

Psychological Dysfunction

The psychological problems pertinent at treatment level two involve self-management deficits. Self-management skills include coping, stress inoculation, critical incidents, time management and self-control. At treatment level two, specific values and interests are cultivated to take the place of drug-related activity.

Coping Skills

The Coping Skills Model described by Monti, Abrams, Kadden and Cooney is useful in guiding occupational therapy sessions.[22] This model presents a variety of coping skill topics that follow a format of providing rationales for each skill, delineating guidelines for skill implementation, practicing each skill, providing handouts and assigning homework. Topics include managing cravings, refusing drinks, planning for emergencies, etc. Stoffel described the effective use of these materials in the occupational therapy treatment program for an adult with alcohol dependence.[23]

Managing stress is an important coping skill that involves integrating artificial dichotomies, achieving relaxation and reducing fears. Coping by integrating dichotomous behaviors is understood when recalling PDS principles. Substance abusers often display a limited behavioral repertoire, characterized by behavioral extremes. For example, the substance abuser might respond in either an aggressive or passive manner, but rarely produces behavior somewhere in between these two polarities.

Kelley's fixed-role therapy is one method of broadening the substance abuser's behavioral repertoire.[15, 24] Fixed role therapy requires the substance abuser to describe the self when using drugs and when sober. Often, the descriptions embody two extremes of behavior. For instance, the addictive self is fun loving, gregarious and outgoing compared to the sober self who is boring, retiring and shy. The substance abuser is asked to combine the best aspects of both selves into a third self or set of role behaviors. Encouragement is given to act out this new role. Feedback helps to determine how well the new role "fits." This role is then modified to enhance comfort with the new behaviors.

Another coping process involves relaxation. Relaxation techniques, ie. biofeedback, progressive relaxation, deep breathing, meditation and self-commands, were discussed earlier as treatment level one methods to control detoxification discomfort. The techniques are the same for treatment level two, but the emphasis changes to issues of generalization and discrimination. The substance abuser generalizes relaxation techniques to a variety of situations thereby enhancing problem solving and improving physical health. Discrimination involves determining the most appropriate relaxation strategy within a given a set of specific circumstances. For example, using progressive relaxation in a time of crisis that demands immediate action is not acceptable. Instead, the substance abuser utilizes deep breathing and self-commands ("easy does it," "stay calm," or "this too shall pass").

Coping training incorporates fear reduction procedures including systematic desensitization and behavioral rehearsal.[25] Systematic desensitization operates on the premise that fear and relaxation cannot be exhibited simultaneously. The substance abuser learns to relax during progressively stressful situations. In those cases where the stressful situation is an anticipated one, the substance abuser, through role playing, rehearses behavioral strategies prior to the stressor's occurrence.

Stress Inoculation

Stress inoculation modifies a person's reactions to stress and controls anger through a three phase process.[18,26,27] The first phase promotes understanding about the physiological aspects of fight or flight reactions. During the second phase, the substance abuser rehearses relaxation techniques in order to control physiological arousal. The self-statements that habitually occupy the individual during stress are changed through cognitive restructuring. In the third phase, the substance abuser is given the opportunity to practice coping skills during exposure to a variety of stressors.

Critical Incidents

The substance abuser's handling of critical incidents or difficult situations is a crucial aspect in developing self-control over drug use.[20] The substance abuser examines self-statements that occur immediately after critical incidents. Short-circuiting ideas (eg. "This shouldn't happen," or "Why did this happen to me") are replaced with statements of capability (eg. "I can handle this situation"). After instituting covert expressions of problem-solving capability, the substance abuser takes charge of the situation. For example, if feeling panicked, the substance abuser presents the outward appearance of being calm (eg. the AA motto: "Fake it until you make it").

Implementing behavioral strategies to cope with the situation is followed by covertly expressing belief in the personal control exercised in the situation. There is appreciation of the choices made in selecting a coping strategy.[20] The substance abuser states covertly, for instance, "I can handle demanding customers and I like the way I responded in a firm, assertive manner."

Time Management

Disrupting old habit patterns as a treatment level two method is differentiated from a similar strategy initiated during treatment level one. The therapist during treatment level one disrupted the substance abuser's old maladaptive habit patterns by providing a schedule that excluded drug-related activities. The substance abuser provided input into this schedule, but primary control over schedule determination was maintained by the therapist. In contrast, treatment level two habit disruption techniques increase the substance abuser's awareness of the situational determinants of addiction. The substance abuser analyzes daily routines with an eye for eliminating those habits that inadvertently perpetuate old, maladaptive behaviors.

Methods of disrupting previous drug-related habit patterns include practicing the opposite, substituting alternative activities, disrupting typical social activities and attendance at AA/NA meetings.[15] Practicing the opposite reorganizes simple, routine activities (eg. changing the route one takes to work) in order to stimulate awareness of habitual ways of approaching and responding to normal events.

In terms of substituting activities, the substance abuser seeks out alternative activities that do not involve drugs or drug-related environments. For example, a substance abuser that enjoys playing baseball discovers that drinking beer during and after the game is a part of the activity. Therefore, the substance abuser joins a church sponsored baseball team where drinking is not involved.

Disrupting social activities is a similar concept to substituting activities and involves staying away from previous drinking or drug "buddies." Attending AA/NA meetings is an obvious method of changing habits as the AA lifestyle, depending on level of involvement, can provide a range of possible substitute activities for drug-related activities.

Self-Control

The concept of self-control seems incongruent with behavioral approaches, but is, in fact, an aspect of learning theory. According to Mosey, an individual has self-control in a given situation when one "alters the frequency of some performance in his own repertoire."[2] Self-control is important because it is difficult to rely on others to reinforce adaptive behaviors. The substance abuser cannot expect others always to provide external control in order to remain abstinent. The goal of treatment level two is to foster internal control.

Self-control occurs when the individual verbally pairs, through self-talk, future behavior with potentially aversive or positive consequences. Self-talk acts as the reinforcing stimulus for increasing adaptive behaviors. Control over behavior results when covertly pairing a stimulus event with the consequences of responding in an adaptive manner.[2] Adaptive behavior must be a powerful motivator in order for the response to be positively influenced.

Helping the substance abuser develop self-control involves identifying the stimulus event, such as an acquaintance offering the substance abuser a drink at a party. Once identified, consequences are defined related to the substance abuser's need system. For instance, "I need to refuse the drink because I cannot stay married and be an effective parent when I'm drunk." To give additional power to the consequences, the therapist helps the substance abuser recall similar circumstances when adaptive behavior was produced with corresponding positive consequences. "At the last party that I avoided drinking, I had a good time talking with friends and dancing with my wife."

Following the addiction through is a technique described by Wallace that is another aspect of the self-control process.[15, 28] The substance abuser imagines an entire drug-related episode, including positive and negative consequences. The substance abuser copes with the desire to use drugs by shifting thinking beyond the initial positive expectations attributed to drug use to the probable delayed consequences. The substance abuser acknowledges that drugs will initially create feelings of relaxation, but that once sober, the old problems will reoccur in addition to new difficulties directly attributable to intoxication.

Values and Interests

Treatment level one focused on enhancing the value of sober behavior. Treatment level two changes the value orientation slightly to include valuing adaptive coping behaviors in place of valuing the short-term consequences of drugs. Values related to appreciation of adaptive behavior are promoted through remediation of specific occupational performance areas.

Treatment level two develops the potential interests identified during treatment level one. The substance abuser develops competence in skill performance. Interests are scheduled into a habit pattern that fills the void left by abstinence from drugs. Engaging in interests becomes a coping strategy to prevent relapse, to replace the enjoyment originally attributed to drugs, to increase social interaction, and to serve as an outlet for negative emotions and tension. Craft groups, activity groups and leisure groups are appropriate treatment methods to accomplish this objective.

Social Dysfunction

Social or interpersonal skills weaken overreliance on the PDS. Social skills training is therefore important for recovery. Consistent failure in interpersonal situations increases the likelihood that sober addicts will return to abusive drug use in order to escape from negative experiences.[29] Methods for social skills training incorporate the typical behavioral strategies of modeling, role-playing, social reinforcement (praise or approval) and transfer training.[30-32]

Structured Learning Therapy, an approach for social skills training, focuses on a variety of skills that range in level of complexity from initiating a conversation to dealing with criticism.[32] Depending on current situational needs, the therapist and the substance abuser select the social skills to be learned. Transfer of training involves homework assignments or real life skill practice. The likelihood that skills are used independently is thus increased.

Assertiveness training is another appropriate social skills intervention for substance abusers. According to Miller, there is an inverse relationship between drug use and assertiveness, ie. the less assertive the substance abuser, the more drugs are likely to be used.[33] Assertiveness training includes the typical skill development strategies of modeling, role playing, feedback, practicing and transfer of training. The cognitive aspects of assertiveness training involve recognizing the differences between aggression, assertion and passivity.[34] The substance abuser discriminates between situations requiring the exercise of personal rights and those involving respect for the rights of others.

Identifying personal goals for assertive interactions strengthens commitment to skill usage. The removal of cognitive and emotional barriers that interfere with actual production of assertive behavior is important. For instance, many addicted women are socialized to believe that "one must always think of others first." Cognitive and affective obstacles to assertiveness are removed through the process of cognitive restructuring.

The substance abuser is also trained in general communication skills. The substance abuser learns the role of nonverbal communication in sending wanted or unwanted messages to others. The substance abuser analyzes personal nonverbal communication, interprets the information being communicated, and ascertains the congruence of the nonverbal message with the verbal content of the communication. The substance abuser focuses on communicating clearly in order to avoid misunderstandings.

It is necessary to teach the substance abuser to change indirect methods of communicating feelings, ideas or values to more direct methods by utilizing "I" messages. Listening skills are another important emphasis, especially given the fact that substance abusers routinely protect themselves with maladaptive defense mechanisms to avoid hearing the "truth" about themselves. Communication also involves a cognitive component. Effective communication is dependent upon the substance abuser's ability to examine assumptions and beliefs formulated about the verbal interaction.[35]

Work Dysfunction

Vocational and Educational Activities

Addressing dysfunctions in the occupational performance area of work is dependent upon whether the substance abuser is currently unemployed, but has had past work experience; is currently employed; or has never been employed outside of the home. Often, the substance abuser entered treatment on threat of losing employment, so that return to work is dependent upon successful rehabilitation. Another common situation is the substance abuser who is unhappy in his or her current job, but has not attempted to make changes.

In terms of education as an occupational performance area requiring intervention, many substance abusers have experienced multiple school failures in the past, often due to attention deficit-hyperactive disorder.[36] Returning to school to obtain a General Education Degree (GED), to complete career objectives or to pursue a new career may be a frightening proposition. School is a major issue in the treatment of adolescent drug abusers and for young adults currently in college.

Occupational therapists develop referral networks that access community resources available for assisting individuals with specific vocational and career problems. Substance abusers require the services of vocational counselors to explore alternative career options, assess their aptitudes for a specific vocation, learn about available training programs, or access financial aid in order to fund education and/or training. The occupational therapist determines which substance abusers could benefit from vocational rehabilitation.

Prevocational skills training is appropriate for those substance abusers who are not ready for vocational rehabilitation. A behavioral approach is an effective method of conducting prevocational skills training for substance abusers who have never been employed, who are undersocialized ("skid row" type), or who have suffered permanent cognitive impairment as a result of chronic drug use. Mosey lists typical prevocational skills that occupational therapy groups address: following written and oral directions, sustaining attention to work tasks, organizing tasks according to priority, performing tasks in an allotted time period, returning to work when interrupted, planning work, giving assistance to others, responding to feedback, etc.[2, 37]

Some substance abusers came into treatment after losing their jobs or they lost their jobs while receiving treatment. For these substance abusers, job search skills need emphasis. Often it has been a long time since the person has had to look for a job. The substance abuser learns how to write a resumé, select potential jobs requiring compatible skills, prepare a cover letter, fill out an application, respond to interview questions, etc. The substance abuser is prepared to answer interview questions regarding the hospitalization for drug addiction. The substance abuser determines the best method for responding to this type of questioning on an application form. The substance abuser must be made aware that the American Disabilities Act offers protection for him or her from job discrimination as long as sobriety is maintained.[23]

There are two issues that substance abusers may face when returning to work. One problem involves returning to an occupation where there is high risk for continued substance abuse, eg. entertainment, business, sales, bartending, etc. Because there is a high risk for relapse, considering a career change is important. This strategy, however, runs the risk of creating intolerable stress related to job changes. When job changes are not possible or advisable, specific coping strategies to deal with tempting situations are developed. For example, a substance abuser who is expected to entertain clients as a method of enabling sales explores entertainment options that do not involve alcohol. If alcohol cannot be avoided, then the substance abuser could carry a glass of ginger ale or attend parties with a coworker who knows the situation.

The other return-to-work issue relates to correcting past poor job performances. Due to a decline in function with the advent of chronic drug use, many problems were created on the job. Often there are coworkers who resent years of covering for the substance abuser. Covering involved completing the substance abuser's work, creating excuses or experiencing constant disappointments for the many times the substance abuser did not follow through as promised. These fellow employees had many hours of extra work as a result of the substance abuser's high rate of absenteeism. The substance abuser is prepared to rectify these wrongs through offering apologies, understanding initial suspiciousness regarding ability to change, and implementing strategies to regain trust.

Home Management

Due to the gradual deteriorating responsibility displayed by the substance abuser, the nonaddicted marriage partner assumed the household duties. Relieving the substance abuser of responsibility is referred to as enabling.[36] With the advent of recovery, the substance abuser and the spouse review current home management roles. Issues are raised when revising the old family structure previously organized around addiction. The spouse initially does not trust the substance abuser, especially after years of the substance abuser failing to follow through with promises. The spouse does not want to give up independence gained as the result of making all the major household decisions. After many years of handling situations without help, it is frustrating to consult with another person. This change in family roles creates many resentments that need discussion. Behavioral and cognitive approaches are utilized to teach both the substance abuser and the family members how to identify and resolve these conflicts about running the household.

Home management difficulties are also experienced by substance abusers faced with divorce. In the past, the substance abuser was dependent upon others to run the household. For these divorced substance abusers, specific home management skills need development.

Many substance abusers have financial difficulties. Chronic drug use aggravated financial problems due to multiple job failures, chronic unemployment, careless financial planning and management, multiple health problems, poor judgment regarding spending, and purchasing the drug supply prior to meeting other financial obligations. Money management training relieves the stress of sobriety. It is difficult to remain sober in the face of severe financial trouble, especially when solutions appear hopeless. Worrying about debt when sober is not an attractive alternative compared to escaping the problem through drug use. As an adjunct to the money management training, the occupational therapist enlists the help of community resources that offer financial counseling.

Care of Others

Care of others in terms of parenting is an important treatment focus. A central theme in the literature on children of alcoholics (CoAs) is the atmosphere of unpredictability and inconsistency found in the substance abuser's home.[39] Typically, while one parent compulsively pursued addiction and characteristically displays denial and violent mood swings, the other parent is primarily concerned with survival. The nonaddicted parent has neither time nor energy to emotionally support the children. As a result, children are confused by the different moods they observe as the addicted parent fluctuates from sobriety to drug-induced psychological states.[40] Morehouse also reported that children tend to blame themselves for their parents' drug use.[40] Confusion is compounded by the role reversal that children of substance abusers often experience.[39] As a consequence of the role reversal, children take the part of the parent, such as cleaning the house, taking care of younger children and taking care of the parent when using.

It cannot be assumed that once the substance abuser recovers, the family dynamics will improve. Addicted parents play a major role in influencing the drug use behavior of their children.[41] Failing to resolve the problems created by dysfunctional parenting, perpetuates drug use to future generations.[42] Occupational therapists teach parenting skills to the substance abuser and, if possible, to the nonaddicted parent as well. The substance abuser becomes aware of possible resentments from the children created by attempts to be a parent after years of neglect or role reversal. The substance abuser carefully and slowly makes positive changes in the relationships with the children. A parenting skills group addresses appropriate behavioral expectations for children, discipline, education, spending time with children, imparting values and morals, etc. [37]

Leisure Dysfunction

The occupational therapist's role in remedying this problem area varies depending upon availability of recreational therapist's. Prior to treatment, the substance abuser's leisure was dependent upon alcohol and other drugs. During initial abstinence, the substance abuser is suddenly devoid of leisure opportunities and often feels that life is no longer enjoyable. It is difficult for the substance abuser to return to previous leisure pursuits as these activities stimulate memories of drug use episodes. Relapse occurs when memories, combined with contextual cues in the environment, overwhelm the substance abuser, resulting in a physiological response experienced as craving.[43] The paradox is that substance abusers must learn how to fill their time previously utilized in drinking or drug use, while realizing that certain activities may stimulate desire for alcohol and drugs.

The goal of leisure skills training is identifying interests not associated with drugs or using environments. Activity functions as a substitute for drug use by producing enjoyment previously attributed exclusively to drug use. It is not uncommon to hear reports from spouses that the substance abuser, prior to treatment, would never go anywhere unless alcohol or drugs were available. Certain leisure activities are strongly connected with drinking by society in general (golf's 19th hole or the bar in the bowling alley). These activities may have to be avoided when planning the substance abuser's new activity routine.

Relapse Prevention

The occupational therapist at treatment level two teaches specific skills related to relapse prevention. Relapse prevention is incorporated into all aspects of the occupational therapy treatment program. Right from the beginning of treatment level two, the occupational therapist and the substance abuser determine the skills necessary for successful coping in the expected or home environment.

Relapse Variables

One of the variables of relapse is post-treatment environmental stressors.[44,45] Therefore, the newly learned coping strategies are all methods of relapse prevention. In order to carry out the cognitive choice to abstain, an individual must also believe in ability to use coping skills as alternatives to drug use. Effective coping leads to a sense of personal control and growing mastery over situations that normally precipitate a relapse. Actual mastery of social skills enhances belief in self-efficacy.[43]

Another relapse variable is drug cue exposure.[46] Drug cues are those objects in the environment that trigger memories of alcohol and other drugs being able to produce positive affect or remove negative affect. The memories, if strong enough, also invoke a physiological response experienced as "craving." Figure 6-5 organizes the concepts of positive and negative reinforcement, dependence, and cue susceptibility in terms of impact on continued drug use. The schematic illustrates how reinforcement effects and contextual cues may, singly or in combination, precipitate reactions that maintain abusive drug use. A different pattern of relapse responses emerges depending on the circuit activated, ie. positive reinforcement, negative reinforcement or contextual cues. These responses generally involve urges to consume the drug, positive outcome expectations for drug use and physiological activation.

Consider, for example, that negative reinforcement is the precipitant. In other words, the person is experiencing a negative affect such as sadness or depression. Triggered outcome expectations include the belief that the drug will relieve the distress. Withdrawal symptoms or arousal associated with avoidance/escape motivation are the specific physiological responses. In contrast, the outcome expectations for a precipitant involving positive reinforcement includes anticipation of pleasurable experiences. Some examples of pleasurable expectations are disinhibition and increases in perceived dominance. Physiological responses involve anticipation of pleasure or reward.

Relapse Avoidance Techniques

Occupational therapists assess the substance abuser's environment through interviews that examine situational circumstances surrounding the typical episode of substance abuse. These microenvironmental influences of drug use include the physical setting, whether a person is alone or with other people, and, if with other people, the degree to which they encourage or

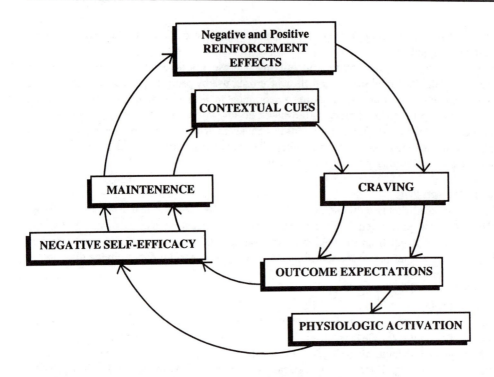

Figure 6-5. Model of dependence.

discourage drug use.[47] Availability of alcohol and drugs along with the conduciveness of the environment to drug use are other contextual considerations.

Evaluation also ascertains the substance abuser's positive and negative incentives that are sources of the positive and negative affect experienced. The substance abuser may, for instance, have an inadequate number of positive incentives or goals to pursue, the goals may be unrealistic (ie. too grandiose or too perfectionistic) or they may be inappropriate.[48,49] Sometimes these goals conflict with other positive goals, thereby making goal attainment unlikely. Furthermore, the substance abuser's life may be overwhelmed by aversive incentives and, as a result, the substance abuser is unable to make progress toward removing these noxious elements.

By assessing the influence of the substance abuser's contextual environment as well as the positive and negative incentives, an accurate picture of coping skill requirements is developed. The substance abuser learns to obtain alternative sources of emotional satisfaction. If there is no other method of pursuing positive feelings, the sober addict eventually remembers how good it felt to use drugs and then begins to use substances again. In this case, the nonchemical incentives produced by goal-seeking did not provide emotional satisfaction that could compete adequately with the good feelings seemingly attainable from drug use.

Occupational therapy treatment techniques emphasize nonchemical incentives. The substance abuser finds sources of satisfaction and avoids unnecessary frustration. Developing a meaningful life without drugs is the key. Treatment involves teaching the substance abuser to avoid, when possible, contextual situations that potentiate craving and tax self-efficacy regarding ability to employ alternative coping methods. The substance abuser is aided in identifying negative affect and connecting feelings to lack of goal fulfillment or to unsatisfying, noxious experiences. The therapist also teaches alternative coping styles, such as anger management or assertiveness, that rid the substance abuser of negative affect and increase the likelihood of goal attainment.

Coping skills training may be ineffective for some substance abusers, however, due to the disruption of these skills by the presence of conditioned cues in the environment. Substance abusers who react strongly to the presence of cues prior to the end of treatment use more of the substance after leaving treatment.[50] Treatment designed to decrease the strength of cue reactivity and the disruptive effects on coping behavior is beneficial. Extinction could be employed for this purpose. Similarities in approach can be drawn from the obsessive-compulsive and phobic disorder treatment literature.[51,52]

Treatment involves presenting the substance abuser with a stimulus (eg. an environment similar to one in which the alcoholic drank, such as a baseball game) in order to elicit the conditioned response. The substance abuser's usual behavior triggered by the stimulus (eg. escape/avoidance or memories of positive affect) is prevented, thus extinguishing the cue response. Prevention of the conditioned response is accomplished by coaching the substance abuser to produce an adaptive response instead of the drug-cued behavior. It is impossible to emit maladaptive behaviors simultaneously with appropriate behavioral responses. For example, at the baseball game, the substance abuser utilizes the strategy of "following the addiction through" when becoming aware of pleasant memories regarding drinking. Even though remembering that the game seemed more enjoyable when drunk, the substance abuser also focuses on the time when he was removed from the game forceably for drunken and disorderly conduct.

This approach is difficult to employ due to lack of research indicating when extinction of cue reactivity should begin in treatment, the frequency of stimulus presentation needed, the strength of the stimulus required, and the exact procedure for identifying relevant cues. Regardless of these problems, occupational therapists should explore the merits of this process further.

Aftercare Planning

The aftercare program continues where treatment level two ended, and is therefore less intensive than the level two inpatient or outpatient program. Aftercare programs design effective coping schedules to be employed independently at home. Coping schedules include a balance of work, self-care and leisure activities. Peak stress times are identified so that coping strategies are incorporated into the schedule at propitious times. For example, the substance abuser might identify that mornings at work are extremely stressful. An aerobics class could be scheduled over the lunch hour to decrease tension. Opportunities for the substance abuser to practice some of the coping strategies outside of the treatment environment are provided. For instance, the substance abuser and family spend a day together in various activities for the purpose of improving relationships. In the aftercare program, the substance abuser reports back how the day went. Effective aftercare planning contributes to decreased recidivism.

Aftercare provides security initially needed to face the stressors and the contextual cues of the expected environment. In conjunction with the substance abuser and the occupational therapist, the aftercare program is delineated prior to discharge from inpatient settings or prior to the scaling down of outpatient services. The aftercare plan describes the goals and methods of treatment level three.

◆ OCCUPATIONAL THERAPY GROUPS ◆

Occupational therapy groups designed for treatment level two foster development of internal control. Specific coping strategies deliberately weaken reliance upon the PDS and are enhanced by a supportive, safe environment. Group formats include one type of developmental group and more advanced thematic groups (Table 6-2). The developmental group specifically involved is the egocentric-cooperative group.

EGOCENTRIC-COOPERATIVE GROUPS

One of the differences between this group type and the project group is the ability to participate in longer-term projects. [37] Another difference is that group members meet the needs of the individual. The therapist subtly directs this process. The therapist also deemphasizes the leadership role that was necessary for the project group. The group functions independently as possible.

The group learns how to select, plan and implement a long-term task through shared interaction. The primary purpose of the group, however, is to learn group normative behaviors.[37] Members are assisted in appropriately requesting that their needs be met by others, particularly needs for recognition. Reinforcement and feedback regarding attempts to obtain appropriate need satisfaction are offered by the therapist and group members.

An example of an egocentric-cooperative group is the publishing of a newspaper. The task is ongoing and long-term, one in fact that continues as new members join and older members leave. Another appropriate long-term task includes selecting, planning and implementing leisure activities for a period of several weeks. The group could function as a patient/client planning council. Egocentric-cooperative groups may be developed for the purpose of preparing a weekly meal. The tasks for the meal involve selecting menus, preparing shopping lists within budget, purchasing food, cooking, cleanup, etc.

As can be seen, some of the same tasks of an egocentric-cooperative group may be utilized in a level one project group. The tasks at the egocentric-cooperative group level are differentiated from the project group by the ongoing, long-term nature of the activity, the change in leadership from therapist to group members, and the emphasis upon utilizing group interactions to meet the needs of fellow group members. Obviously, then, there will be times when the group needs to discuss the behavior of group members, the feelings produced, and the methods in which needs were met by each other.

Additionally, to ensure that the substance abuser can transfer this learning to the home situation, the group addresses application to the "real world." The group examines ways to obtain need-satisfying group interactions. The substance abuser is encouraged to identify group membership possibilities that offer similar experiences. Examples of group experiences obtainable from the community are AA/NA groups or other self-help groups, professional associations, church groups, leisure- or hobby-related groups, arts groups, etc.

THEMATIC GROUPS

Higher level thematic groups are important at this treatment level in teaching coping skills that weaken reliance upon the PDS. Skills training may focus on the performance components or the occupational performance skills related to work and leisure activities.

Social Skills Training Groups

Social skills groups are important for recovery. Consistent failure in interpersonal situations increases the likelihood that sober addicts will return to abusive drug use in order to escape from these negative experiences. Social skills groups and assertiveness training groups improve ability in employing nonverbal expressions (eg. eye contact), refusing unreasonable requests,

Table 6-2
Treatment Level Two Groups

Groups	Factors to be Considered with Substance Abusers	Strategies
Egocentric-Cooperative Group	Development of long-term relationships and feelings of belonging	Meal preparation Leisure planning Group craft projects Unit newspaper Council
Thematic Group	Level two skill needs of the treatment population	Assertiveness training Anger management Communication Problem-solving Occupational performance

making difficult requests, expressing feelings, responding to criticism and initiating conversations. Assertiveness training groups also strengthen the substance abusers ability to refuse drugs or alcohol in a social situation.

Research consistently shows that behavioral methods (ie. modeling, coaching, role-playing, behavioral rehearsal and homework assignments) are superior over traditional supportive social skills training (didactic lecture and discussions) in teaching assertiveness skills to substance abusers.[53-56] Group methods of social and assertiveness skills training are more effective than individual behavioral training methods and individual traditional supportive approaches.[57] In addition to having a positive impact upon length of time remaining abstinent, research also indicates that assertiveness training for substance abusers is an effective method for improving vocational and interpersonal skill competency.[53,54]

Problem-Solving Groups

Problem-solving groups focus on skills that enhance problem solving and that remediate the typical deficit cognitive components. Problem-solving includes the ability to define problems in terms of a need rather than in terms of a premature problem solution.[58] For example, "I need to resolve my feelings of anger toward my spouse" versus "I am avoiding my wife because I'm angry."

Another strategy involves evaluating the cause of the problem as being outside the self (eg. death of a loved one), a habitual behavior pattern (eg. drinking nightly after work), or a maladaptive thought pattern (eg. believing that drugs are effective in relieving tension). The tendency to define problems as a result of personality deficits is thus extinguished. When problems are attributed to personality flaws (eg. "I drink because I am weak"), problem-solving is stifled.

Problem-solving groups therefore not only focus on behavioral skills, but also emphasize realistic belief in ability to solve problems. Real problems drawn from the experience of group members demonstrate effectiveness of the behavioral and cognitive restructuring approaches. Group members assist each other in implementing the behavioral steps as well as in confronting the maladaptive cognitive beliefs interfering with problem solution effectiveness.

Anger Management Groups

Persons having difficulty managing anger are taught to cope with situations that in the past triggered a maladaptive anger response. Skill in managing anger is an appropriate theme for occupational therapy groups. In fact, Taylor described a group treatment strategy that consists of six stages.[59]

During the first stage of anger treatment, group members learn about the relationship between stress and anger, the components of anger and the use of anger to cue stress management behaviors. The second stage of treatment increases awareness of personal levels of arousal, cognitions, environment and behaviors typical of anger episodes. The third stage uses modeling to demonstrate adaptive coping responses to stressful situations. During the fourth stage, group members practice these newly learned adaptive coping skills. The fifth stage utilizes feedback to augment performance. The sixth stage assigns homework that demands independent practice of coping techniques in real-life situations.

Taylor describes specific coping skills for changing physiological arousal, cognitive processing, environmental stimuli and behavioral reactions associated with anger.[59] Physiological arousal control uses relaxation techniques, such as progressive relaxation, relaxation imagery and deep breathing cued relaxation.[60] Once developed, these coping skills are applied to anger arousing imagery within sessions and to angering situations between sessions.

Cognitive modification involves identifying cognitions that contribute to anger.[59] More adaptive cognitions are then developed that reduce anger. Exploration of past angry episodes helps identify commonalities related to typical environmental stimuli. Problem-solving occurs regarding managing this stimuli more effectively or changing environmental circumstances. Finally, remediating skill deficits related to communication, social interaction, time management, parenting and problem solving may prevent current inappropriate behavioral responses to anger.

◆ REEVALUATION ◆

Determining readiness for treatment level three is dependent upon reevaluation of progress toward treatment level two goals. Improvement in coping ability and application of these techniques to occupational performance areas of work and leisure demonstrate improvement. Responsibility in maintaining abstinence and internal control regarding ability to make effective changes indicate significant treatment level two progress. Informal and formal strategies are utilized in reevaluation, giving preference to tools capable of test-retest comparisons. Documenting progress illustrates the medical necessity of occupational therapy. Lack of progress may indicate need to redesign the treatment plan or need to revert back to treatment level one strategies.

◆ CONCLUSIONS ◆

Frames of reference consistent with the issues of treatment level two were identified and described. Action-consequence, cognitive-behavioral and the model of human occupation are three approaches that employ supportive therapeutic styles in the teaching of coping strategies that weaken reliance on the PDS. The specific drug abused determines the coping strategies to be learned.

Emphasis in treatment is placed on the cognitive skills of generalization, discrimination, problem-solving and challenging irrational thoughts. Self-management is improved after learning alternative coping strategies, applying the principles of stress inoculation, dealing with critical incidents, managing time and implementing self-control. Valuing coping abilities and selecting interests that assist coping are also important. Social skills training and addressing work or leisure related performance dysfunctions were highlighted.

Treatment level two groups teach alternative coping skills that weaken reliance upon maladaptive coping mechanisms. A supportive group approach is necessary to foster internal control. Egocentric-cooperative groups and higher level thematic groups are appropriate. Reevaluation assesses progress toward independence in coping, ability to prevent relapse and assumption of responsibility.

References

1. American Occupational Therapy Association Uniform Terminology Task Force: Uniform terminology for occupational therapy (2nd ed.). *Am J Occup Ther* 43(12): 808-815, 1989.
2. Mosey AC: *Three Frames of Reference for Mental Health*. Thorofare, NJ: Slack Inc., 1970, p. 91.
3. Bruce MA, Borg B: *Frames of Reference in Psychosocial Occupational Therapy*. Thorofare, NJ: Slack Inc., 1987.
4. D'Zurilla TJ: *Problem-Solving Therapy: A Social Competence Approach to Clinical Intervention*. New York: Springer Publishing Co., 1986.
5. Cubie SH, Kaplan KL, Kielhofner G: Program development. In Kielhofner G (Ed.): *A Model of Human Occupation: Theory and Application*. Baltimore, MD: Williams & Wilkins, 1985, pp. 156-167.
6. Kielhofner G (Ed): *A Model of Human Occupation: Theory and Application*. Baltimore, MD: Williams and Wilkins, 1985.
7. Carver CS, Scheier MF, Weintraub JK: Assessing coping strategies: A theoretically based approach. *J Pers Soc Psychol* 56(2): 267-283, 1989.
8. Gambrill ED, Richey C: An assertion inventory for use in assessment and research. *Behav Ther* 6: 550-561, 1975.
9. Hawkins JD, Catalano RF, Wells EA: Measuring effects of a skills training intervention for drug abusers. *J Consult Clin Psychol* 54(5): 661-664, 1986.
10. Heppner PP, Petersen CH: The development and implications of a personal problem-solving inventory. *J Counsel Psychol* 29: 66-75, 1982.
11. Rotter JB: Generalized expectancies for internal vs. external control of reinforcement. *Psychol Monograph 8* (Whole No. 609): 1-28, 1966.
12. Kaplan H, Sadock B: *Comprehensive Textbook—Modern Synopsis of Psychiatry III* (4th ed). Baltimore, MD: Williams & Wilkins, 1988.
13. Toglia JP: Generalization of treatment: A multicontext approach to cognitive perceptual impairment in adults with brain injury. *Am J Occup Ther* 45(6): 505-516, 1991.
14. Abreu BC, Toglia JP: Cognitive rehabilitation: A model for occupational therapy. *Am J Occup Ther* 41(7): 439-448, 1987.
15. Wallace J: Behavioral modification methods as adjuncts to psychotherapy. In Zimberg S, Wallace J, and Blume SB (Eds.): *Practical Approaches to Alcoholism Psychotherapy* (2nd ed.). New York: Plenum Press, 1985, pp. 112-115, 110-112.
16. Perls FS: *Gestalt Therapy Verbatim*. Lafayette, Los Angeles: Real People Press, 1969.
17. Beck AT, Rush AJ, Shaw BF, Emery G: *Cognitive Therapy of Depression*. New York: Guilford Press, 1979.
18. Meichenbaum D: *Cognitive-behavior Modification*. New York: Plenum Press, 1977.
19. Ellis A: *Reason and Emotion in Psychotherapy*. New York: Lyle Stuart, 1962.
20. Emery G, Hollon SD, Bedrosian RC: *New Directions in Cognitive Therapy a Casebook*. New York: The Guilford Press, 1981.
21. Beck AT: Cognitive therapy: Nature and relation to behavior therapy. *Behav Ther* 1: 184-200, 1970.
22. Monti PM, Abrams DB, Kadden RM, Cooney NL: *Treating Alcohol Dependence: A Coping Skills Training Guide*. New York: Guilford Press, 1989.
23. Stoffel VC: The Americans With Disabilities Act of 1990 as applied to an adult with alcohol dependence. *Am J Occup Ther* 46(7): 640-644, 1992.
24. Kelley JR: *The Psychology of Personal Constructs* Vols. I and II. New York: Norton, 1955.
25. Cautela JR: Treatment of compulsive behavior by covert sensitization. *Psychol Rec* 16: 33-41, 1966.
26. Novaco R: Anger Control: *The Development and Evaluation of an Experimental Treatment*. Lexington, MA: Heath & Co., 1975.
27. Taylor E: Anger intervention. *Am J Occup Ther* 42(3): 147-155, 1988.

28. Lazarus AA: *Behavior Therapy and Beyond*. New York: McGraw-Hill, 1971.

29. Bandura A: *Social Foundations of Thought and Action*. Englewood Cliffs, NJ: Prentice-Hall, 1985.

30. Nickel I: Adapting structured learning therapy for use in a psychiatric adult day hospital. *The Canadian J Occup Ther* 55(1): 21-25, 1988.

31. Goldstein AP, Gershaw NJ, Sprafkin RP: Structured learning therapy: Development and evaluation. *Am J Occup Ther* 33: 635-639, 1979.

32. Lillie MD, Armstrong HE: Contributions to the development of psychoeducational approaches to mental health service. *Am J Occup Ther* 36(7): 438-443, 1982.

33. Miller PM: Behavior therapy in the treatment of alcoholism. In Marlatt GA & Nathan PE (Eds.): *Behavioral Approaches to Alcoholism*. New Brunswick, NJ: Center for Studies on Alcohol, 1978.

34. Lange AJ, Jakubowski P: *Responsible Assertive Behavior*. Springfield, IL: Research Press, 1976.

35. Bolton R: *People Skills*. Englewood Cliffs, NJ: Prentice-Hall, Inc., 1979.

36. Sher KJ, Levenson RW: Risk for alcoholism and individual differences in the stress-response-dampening effect of alcohol. *J Abnorm Psychol* 91: 350-368, 1982.

37. Mosey AC: *Psychosocial Components of Occupational Therapy*. New York: Raven Press, 1986.

38. Whitfield CL: Co-alcoholism: Recognizing a treatable illness. *Fam Comm Health* (August): 16-27, 1984.

39. Nardi PM: Children of alcoholics: A role-theoretical perspective. *J Soc Psychol* 115: 237-245, 1981.

40. Morehouse E: Working in the schools with children of alcoholic parents *Health Soc Work* 4(4): 144-162, 1979.

41. Barnes GM: The development of adolescent drinking behaviors: An evaluative review of the impact of the socialization process within the family. *Adolescence* 12: 571-591, 1977.

42. Russell M, Henderson C, Blume SB: *Children of Alcoholics: A Review of the Literature*. New York: Children of Alcoholics Foundation, 1985.

43. Marlatt GA, Gordon JR: *Relapse Prevention*. New York: Guilford Press, 1985.

44. Finney JW, Moos RH, Mewborn CR: Posttreatment experiences and treatment outcome of alcoholic patients six months and two years after hospitalization. *J Consult Clin Psychol* 48: 17-29, 1980.

45. McLellan AT, Luborsky L, O'Brien CP, Barr HL, Evano F: Alcohol and drug abuse treatment in three different populations: Is there improvement and is it predictable? *Am J Alcohol Abuse* 12: 101-120, 1986.

46. Kaplan RF, Cooney NL, Berker LH, Gillespie RA, Meyer RE, Ponerleau OF: Reactivity to alcohol-related cues: Physiological and subjective responses in alcoholics and nonproblem drinkers. *J Stud Alcohol* 46: 267-272, 1985.

47. McCarty D: Environmental factors in substance abuse: The microsetting. In Galizio M & Maisto SA (Eds.): *Determinants of Substance Abuse: Biological, Psychological, and Environmental Factors*. New York: Plenum Press, 1985, pp. 247-281.

48. Klinger E: *Meaning and Void: Inner Experience and the Incentives in People's Lives*. Minneapolis, MN: University of Minnesota Press, 1977.

49. Klinger E: On the self-management of mood, affect, and attention. In Karoly P & Kanfer F (Eds.): *Self-management and Behavior Change: From Theory to Practice*. Elmsford, NY: Pergamon, 1982, pp. 129-164.

50. Niaura RS, Rohsenow DJ, Binkoff JA, Monti PM, Pedraza M, Abrams DB: Relevance of cue reactivity to understanding alcohol and smoking relapse. *J Abnorm Psychol* 97(2): 133-152, 1988.

51. Foa EB, Kozak MJ: Emotional processing of fear: Exposure to corrective information. *Psychol Bull* 99: 20-35, 1986.

52. Rachman S, Hodgson R: *Obsessions and Compulsions*. Englewood Cliffs, NJ: Prentice-Hall, 1980.

53. Freedburg EJ, Johnston WE: Effects of assertion training within context of a multi-modal alcoholism treatment program for employed alcoholics. *Psychol Rep* 48: 379-386, 1981.

54. Foy DW, et al: Social skills training to improve alcoholics' vocational interpersonal competency. *J Coun Psych* 26(2): 128-132, 1979.

55. Brown LS, Ostrow F: The development of an assertiveness program on an alcoholism unit. *Int J Addict* 15(3): 323-327, 1980.

56. Callner DA, Ross SM: The assessment and training of assertive skills with drug addicts: A preliminary study. *Int J Addict* 13(2): 227-239, 1978.

57. Oei T, Jackson P: Long-term effects of group and individual social skills training with alcoholics. *Addict Behav* 5: 129-136, 1980.

58. Mahoney MJ: *Self-change*. New York: WW Norton & Co., 1979.

59. Taylor E: Anger intervention. *Am J Occup Ther* 42(3): 147-155, 1988.

60. Hazaleus SL, Deffenbacher JL: Relaxation and cognitive treatments of anger. *J Consult Clin Psychol* 54(2): 222-226, 1986.

Assessment and Treatment
Level Three

INTRODUCTION

This chapter explores the frames of reference capable of challenging continued usage of the PDS in order for personality growth to occur. Two frames of reference are described and include object relations and model of human occupation. The occupational therapy treatment diagnosis addresses the psychological component dysfunctions that restrict personality growth required for expanded role performance. The psychological issues of addiction are resolved by enhancing self-awareness and ultimately self-actualization.

The substance abuser learns to act on insight, thus developing role performance behaviors consistent with identified values. The occupational therapist employs a confrontational therapeutic style that prevents continued maladaptive defense mechanism usage. Treatment strategies are implemented on an outpatient basis, with the substance abuser primarily responsible for implementing changes within the home environment.

◆ FRAMES OF REFERENCE ◆

Progression to treatment level three indicates that cognitive, social, sensorimotor and occupational performance dysfunctions have been resolved. However, treatment level three monitors maintenance of coping behaviors in occupational roles. The main emphasis of treatment, though, is upon the psychological issues of addiction and the way in which these problems restrict functional performance. A goal of treatment is to enhance self-concept, thereby promoting the personality growth necessary for successful occupational performance. The PDS is confronted in order to discontinue remaining reliance upon maladaptive defense mechanisms. Using healthy values to formulate decisions regarding performance in new or expanded roles is an important treatment concern (Table 7-1).

Two frames of reference meet the criteria described above, including model of human occupation and object relations. Object relations frame of reference challenges PDS utilization by developing insight. Acting on insight modifies behavior in a manner consistent with the requirements of a healthy value structure and new or expanded occupational roles. The model of human occupation focuses on the substance abuser's value structure and new skill development. Utilization of values and skills in healthy role performance is emphasized.

Table 7-1
Level Three Treatment Focus in Two Frames of Reference

Treatment Focus	Object Relations	Model of Human Occupation
Psychological Components Self-expression Self-awareness Self-identity Self-actualization	Symbol production Identify needs Explore unconscious Resolve universal issues (complexes) "Work through"	Improve achievement level: previous interests, personal causation, habits and skills Establish new interests Establish new roles and habits Develop new, complex skills
Values	Value conflicts	Evaluate behavior in terms of value system
Expanded Roles	Reactions to new roles	Develop new roles Refine old roles

PDS Status = Confronted; Treatment Outcome = Personality Development

MODEL OF HUMAN OCCUPATION

The model of human occupation addresses some of the treatment level three problems, but not necessarily those related to insight regarding addiction. This frame of reference promotes growth by helping the substance abuser progress to the achievement level of occupational functioning (Figure 7-1). Achievement involves "striving to maintain and enhance performance in occupations with standards of performance and excellence."[1] Control over behavior results when an individual has developed skills and habits that allow successful interactions with the environment. Achievement is usually required by several roles that an individual assumes in life.

Lack of achievement produces inefficacious occupational performance. Achievement is necessary for replacement of drugs as a source of positive reinforcement. Inefficacy is defined as a "reduction or interference with performance accompanied by dissatisfaction."[1] In other words,

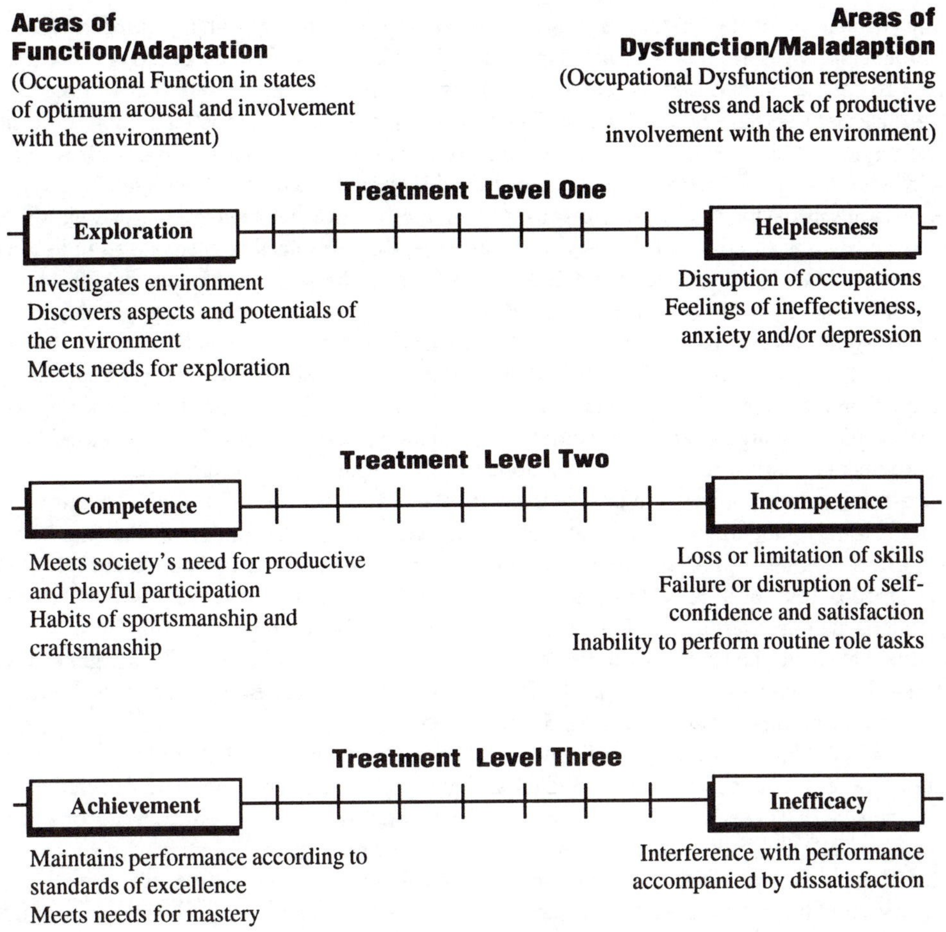

**Areas of
Function/Adaptation**
(Occupational Function in states
of optimum arousal and involvement
with the environment)

**Areas of
Dysfunction/Maladaption**
(Occupational Dysfunction representing
stress and lack of productive
involvement with the environment)

Treatment Level One

| Exploration | | Helplessness |

Investigates environment
Discovers aspects and potentials of
the environment
Meets needs for exploration

Disruption of occupations
Feelings of ineffectiveness,
anxiety and/or depression

Treatment Level Two

| Competence | | Incompetence |

Meets society's need for productive
and playful participation
Habits of sportsmanship and
craftsmanship

Loss or limitation of skills
Failure or disruption of self-
confidence and satisfaction
Inability to perform routine role tasks

Treatment Level Three

| Achievement | | Inefficacy |

Maintains performance according to
standards of excellence
Meets needs for mastery

Interference with performance
accompanied by dissatisfaction

Figure 7-1. Three levels of function-dysfunction continuums in the model of human occupation.

there is "a reduction of personal causation and negative impact on interests, values, roles and habits."[1] Generally, the individual is unable to produce meaningful occupational behavior and as a result, the individual is extremely critical of personal abilities. Lack of pride in occupational behavior may contribute to relapse, such that the substance abuser uses drugs to reduce the negative feelings associated with inefficacy.

OBJECT RELATIONS

According to the object relations frame of reference, persons, environments, activities and media are viewed as objects invested with psychic energy.[2] An individual interacts with these objects in order to satisfy personal needs, to grow and to achieve self-actualization. Some objects enhance personal development while other objects interfere with positive growth and therefore, must be removed.[2]

The person is characterized as a dynamic energy system, containing aspects known (conscious) and aspects unknown (unconscious) to the self.[2] The self is composed of three parts referred to as the id, ego and superego. The id is that portion of the self that is unable to differentiate between reality and fantasy. The ego is responsible for realistically assessing the outside world and as a result determines the nature of one's reality. The superego refers to the conscience or the development of what is considered by society to be good and bad.

A person's behavior is characterized by a dynamic balance between needs, drives, affect, cognitive processes and the will.[2] Needs are inherent predispositions that motivate an individual to sustain life and pursue social activity. According to Maslow, needs are hierarchically arranged, beginning with basic needs and progressing to higher level needs, ie. physiological, safety, love and belonging, esteem and self-actualization.[3] Drives are active efforts by the individual to achieve need satisfaction.[2] Affect consists of emotions and feelings experienced relative to interactions with objects. Cognitive processes refer to the act of perception, representation, and organization of stimuli into memory. The will involves the individual's ability to make choices among available actions for the purpose of satisfying needs.

Relationships with objects are unique and capable of assisting the individual in maximizing potential.[2] Rarely, though, are these interrelationships perfectly balanced. An imbalance between drives, affect, cognitive processes and will produces complexes. Often, complexes are relegated to the unconscious and may be inadvertently expressed through symbol production. An unconscious that is overburdened by complexes can prevent self-actualization. However, the individual can make contact with these unconscious complexes and eventually integrate them back into the conscious self. As the result of this integration, psychic energy tied to the complex is released and becomes available for need satisfaction.

The object relations frame of reference promotes abstinence by challenging the defense structure of the substance abuser.[4] Individual and group psychotherapy facilitate understanding of each substance abuser's total life situation. The substance abuser becomes aware of needs, interpersonal relationships, social and drug use history, and personality strengths and weaknesses. Therapy may be directed to proximal and distal determinants of drug use as well as to secondary conditions produced by substance abuse. Issues produced by abstinence are also addressed.

Proximal conditions are those circumstances that occur in the present, eg. an irate employer. Distal determinants involve conflicts and reality distortions based on early relationships with significant others. Secondary conditions are those that result as a consequence of drug use. This may involve current family and business relationships, sexual dysfunction, financial issues and legal problems. Ceasing drug use when trying to remain sober in the face of stress and other tempting situations may create other problematic conditions requiring individual and group psychotherapy.

◆ OCCUPATIONAL THERAPY DIAGNOSIS ◆

FUNCTIONAL EVALUATION

Not all substance abusers reach treatment level three. This level is not implemented unless the substance abuser possesses the necessary cognitive ability to engage in abstract exploration of life meaning and experience. Coping skills must be of adequate strength to compensate for the pain associated with exploring issues surrounding the addiction. Even though treatment is indicated, some substance abusers elect not to continue with therapy. The door to treatment is left open in case the substance abuser desires professional help in the future.[4]

Some substance abusers do not need extensive personality restructuring. This is particularly true of substance abusers who do not have a family history of addiction, who experienced substance abuse in response to severe stressors, and who developed substance abuse later in life.[5] Pattison determined that approximately 50 percent of the alcoholic population would return to mature levels of personality operation once achieving sobriety.[5]

Data that substantiates treatment level three problems indicate limited insight into the issues surrounding addiction, particularly problems involving self-concept. For example, after an interview, it is apparent that the substance abuser is beginning to express insight into the impact that his father's drinking had on his life. The substance abuser, though, is unable to give clear examples of this influence and it is obvious that resentment toward his father is unresolved. The substance abuser denies this resentment and does not seem aware of the hostile emotions expressed during the interview when discussing his father.

Lack of a crystallized value set or demands from the expected environment for expanded role behaviors are other signals for treatment level three intervention. Expanded role behavior refers to instances where the substance abuser, after treatment, is required to engage in unfamiliar occupational performances as might be the case if returning to a different job, searching for a job or beginning school. These new experiences contribute to a high level of stress that might not be typical if returning to a safe, familiar environment. Lack of a crystallized value set means that the substance abuser has difficulty identifying values and using these values as a guide to decision making.

Measurement tools appropriate for treatment level three evaluation supply data regarding poor self-concept. Determining awareness of values and ability to act on the value structure is another possibility for evaluation focus. The occupational therapist might also evaluate performance in new or expanded roles (Table 7-2). There are a variety of instruments available. Ultimate selection depends upon the information desired and the characteristics of the treatment population.

The Personal Orientation Inventory measures values and behavior important in the development of self-actualization.[6] The Life Purpose Questionnaire (LPQ) determines an individual's sense of life meaning.[7] The Michill Adjective Rating Scale (MARS) consists of 48 adjectives, such as "dominating, nervous, anxious," and utilizes a five-point rating scale ranging from very untypical to very typical.[8] This instrument measures a number of personality traits that could affect maintenance of sobriety, especially when professional help is terminated.

FUNCTIONAL ASSESSMENT

Similar to the other treatment levels, evaluation data are organized into an occupational therapy diagnosis. Treatment planning is based upon data synthesis. The occupational component dysfunction primarily involves psychological issues related to self-concept and self-actualization. Values dysfunction is another component dysfunction commonly addressed. These problems influence engagement in the unfamiliar tasks of new or expanded roles. A sample occupational therapy diagnosis is presented in Figure 7-2.

Functional status, in addition to the occupational therapy diagnosis, includes the functional change and the functional prognosis. The functional change summarizes the progress resulting from treatment level two intervention. Prognosis recognizes the type of progress made prior to treatment level three. Making significant progress in terms of learning coping skills and applying newly learned skills independently indicates a good prognosis. Developing an effective aftercare plan also suggests a good prognosis. Treatment level three evaluation indicating less severe

Table 7-2
Treatment Level Three Evaluations

Frame of Reference	Psychological	Values	Expanded Roles
Object Relations	Azima Battery BH Battery Fidler Battery Goodman Battery Magazine Picture Collage Shoemyen Battery	Projective Techniques Life Purpose Questionnaire (LPQ)	Michill Adjective Rating Scale (MARS)
Model of Human Occupation	Coopersmith Self-Esteem Inventories Tennessee Self-Concept Scale Self-Esteem Scale	Occupational Case Analysis Interview and Rating Scale Occupational Role History The Role Checklist The Salience Inventory The Rokeach Value Survey California Life Goals Evaluation Schedule Personal Orientation Inventory	Adolescent Role Assessment Occupational Role History The Role Checklist The Salience Inventory

Functional Diagnosis

Role Dysfunction	Expresses concern about ability to go to school to pursue a GED. Obtaining a GED is necessary for desired job promotion.
Performance Dysfunction	Has a history of school failure. Low grades contributed to dropping out of high school.
Component Dysfunction	Decreased self-concept regarding academic abilities. Lacks practice and needs standby assist in using newly learned coping skills in dealing with stress at school.
Cues	In the past, used alcohol to cope with failure. Does not ask for help when encountering problems. Score on the Michill Adjective Rating Scale (MARS) suggests possible difficulty in maintaining abstinence.
Pathology	Alcohol dependence.
Functional Change	(after completion of treatment level 2) Successfully uses relaxation and assertiveness techniques on the treatment unit, completes coping skill assignments independently, has incorporated coping and stress management skills into daily routine.
Functional Prognosis	Coping skill success and family and work support for academic goals suggest ability to reach treatment level 3 goals stated in the treatment plan.

Figure 7-2. Occupational therapy treatment level three assessment.

erosion of self-concept, few values conflicts and capability in assuming new roles are predictive of further treatment success. Existence of a strong support system is advantageous as well.

Level three treatment is often not considered necessary by third party payers, especially if treatment appears to be overly focused upon the components of function. Some insurance companies go so far as to clearly state in policy that self-esteem treatment is not reimbursable. There is a tendency for therapists to address self-esteem and other self-concept issues, for example, without making it clear to insurance companies the functional limitations that arise from a psychological component dysfunction. Therefore, a clearly stated functional diagnosis, complete with expectations for specific functional improvements to result within a manageable time frame, is more likely to convince insurance companies of the need for further therapy.

Notice in the occupational therapy diagnosis presented in Figure 7-2 that the emphasis is not upon self-concept, but is upon the substance abuser's difficulty in preparing for increased job responsibilities that require a return to school for more training. The occupational therapist presents this situation as a high risk relapse situation in which the substance abuser lacks preparation.

◆ OCCUPATIONAL THERAPY TREATMENT ◆

CONFRONTATIONAL APPROACH

Progression to treatment level three indicates need for a confrontional style of interaction (Figure 7-3). Insight and resolution of the major issues of addiction are the goals of treatment. In order to identify and face these issues, the therapist confronts behaviors and attitudes signalling unresolved problems. Continued usage of the preferred defense mechanism is also challenged. Confrontation is not a license to insult the self-worth or human dignity of the substance abuser. Compassion and empathy are important aspects of successful confrontation. Challenging the PDS requires specific therapeutic skills including immediacy, concreteness, confrontation and a "total way of being."[9]

Immediacy

Immediacy is an aspect of challenging the substance abuser. The therapist shares with the substance abuser what is "immediately" going on in the therapeutic relationship. The process of connecting the substance abuser with the "here and now" keeps reality in focus.[9] Immediacy is in direct response to the substance abuser's tendency to overuse the defense mechanisms of denial and projection. Denial and projection enable the substance abuser to recreate reality in a way that allows feeling more comfortable, at least temporarily. In the long run, more discomfort is actually produced.

For example, consider a situation in which the therapist is angry with the substance abuser and the occupational therapy group session is generally nonproductive. Perhaps the substance abuser is avoiding a particular issue even though redirected back to it several times by the therapist and other group members. Immediacy occurs when the therapist stops the process and asks what is really happening. Feelings of both the therapist and the substance abuser are brought to the level where they can be dealt with so that the business of therapy can proceed.

Concreteness

Concreteness is "the act of keeping the client's and the therapist's own communications specific, getting to the "whats", "whens", "wheres" and "hows" of relevant concerns."[9] Many times a substance abuser generalizes and skirts around problems as a method of conflict minimization and avoidance. The therapist must be astute at picking up clues regarding the substance abuser's real concerns. A substance abuser might state, for example, that "all husbands and wives have problems." The real meaning may be that the substance abuser's marriage is in trouble.

Confrontation

Another aspect of a challenging therapeutic style is confrontation. This is probably one of the most difficult and most abused therapeutic skills. Therapists err either in not confronting when needed or confronting too much and too soon. Confrontation brings the substance abuser face to face with reality. The substance abuser must be ready for confrontation. Confrontation is indicated when discrepancies exist between: "a) what a substance abuser is saying and the therapist's perception of what he is experiencing, b) what he is saying and what the therapist heard him say at an earlier time, and c) what he is saying now and his actions in his everyday life."[9]

Because confrontation is powerful, the therapist must be careful in deciding when to confront. Confronting too soon may create strong urges to leave treatment and use drugs.

SUPPORTIVE ATTITUDES

Empathy: Focus on behavioral/verbal discrepancies

Genuineness: Challenge ownership of feelings

Respect: "Push" into action; clarify problems and alternative solutions

Self-disclosure: Share emotions

Warmth: Confront self-centered attention and feigned caring

TOTAL WAY OF BEING

Potency: Challenge powerlessness

Self-Actualization: Challenge disregard for potential sources of happiness

CHALLENGING STYLE

Immediacy: Redirect toward issues

Confrontation: Confront behaviors signalling unresolved issues; Avoid insulting self-worth/dignity

Concreteness: Challenge faulty reasoning

Figure 7-3. Treatment level three therapeutic use of self: Confrontive interactive approach.

Guidelines for confrontation involve answering four questions: "1) Will he accept my confrontation as an invitation to explore himself?, 2) Is he open to knowing how he is seen or experienced by others?, 3) Can he tolerate some discomfort and mental pain which may result from my confrontation?, and 4) Does he believe that I care about him?"[9]

It is not important that the therapist might be uncomfortable confronting the substance abuser. The therapist must be able to confront properly when indicated. As a therapist, being too comfortable with confrontation may signal a lack of empathy in the relationship.

Total Way of Being

A total way of being, on the part of the therapist, produces a relationship capable of promoting self-actualization in the substance abuser.[9] Self-actualization is a process, not an outcome, that is important in replacing the positive expectations regarding the effects of drugs. Positive affect resulting from memories of pleasant drinking or drug-use experiences is a powerful component of relapse. Replacing these memories of positive affect with peak experiences generated from "sober" interactions with others is a necessary part of relapse prevention. Having "peak experiences" (moments of ecstasy or spirituality) signal that the self-actualizing process is occurring.

Potency is a component of self-actualizing relationships and refers to the charismatic or magnetic quality of the therapist.[9] The therapist must be capable of communicating a dynamic and an involved attitude toward the substance abuser. The therapist's personal power and enthusiasm helps to motivate the substance abuser. This therapist characteristic is appropriate for the substance abuser's tendency to respond to emotional rather than rational therapy styles.

However, the therapist is careful not to overwhelm the substance abuser with these charismatic qualities. This preference for dynamic interactions was discussed as an aspect of the PDS. The substance abuser generally has difficulty relating to a therapist who has a flat affect and appears uninvolved or disinterested.

TREATMENT PLANNING

As was true of the other two treatment levels, long- and short-term goals are delineated that indicate the assistance levels (ranging from total assistance to independence) achievable by treatment termination. The long-term goals focus on development of skills necessary for expanded role behaviors. Short-term goals identify the underlying psychological and value dysfunctions restricting performance in expanded roles. Writing treatment goals in this manner is another way to facilitate third party reimbursement for services. The goals are clearly functionally based and clarify the relationship between improvements in psychological component functioning and occupational performance functioning.

The substance abuser is an active participant in treatment planning, taking leadership in the process. As indicated in Chapter 6, treatment level three planning is best when conducted prior to discharge from the treatment level two inpatient program or the reduction in frequency of the more intense treatment level two outpatient program. Treatment level three planning is referred to as the aftercare plan. Figure 7-4 outlines sample goals for treatment level three.

Long-term Goals

1. Pt. will independently implement GED study program.
2. Pt. will successfully complete GED program with standby assist (3 months).

Short-term Goals

1. Pt. will independently contact GED program to obtain information (1 week).
2. Pt. will independently analyze daily schedule to determine ability to include GED study and class attendance (1 week).
3. Pt. will independently enroll in GED program (2 weeks).
4. Pt. will independently organize a home-study program to complement class work (3 weeks).
5. Pt. will independently monitor stress signals daily after instituting GED study (3 weeks).
6. Pt. will independently include exercise program two times per week to control GED stress (4 weeks).

Methods

Outpatient Role Exploration Group
Homework assignments
GED course enrollment
Community exercise group

Figure 7-4. Sample treatment level three goals.

STRATEGIES

The occupational therapy treatment strategies at treatment level three address psychological and value dysfunctions. Psychological problems primarily involve a decreased self-concept that interferes with successful role performance. Values dysfunction indicates difficulty in identifying pertinent values necessary for guiding decision making. Treatment strategies additionally focus on new role behaviors that are required by the home environment and that might impact ability to stay sober.

Psychological Dysfunction

Psychological issues are the most pertinent at treatment level three. This treatment level is concerned with the substance abuser's ability to engage in mature relationships that are reflective of appropriate need satisfaction. The substance abuser learns how to satisfy needs and how to remove need-inhibiting barriers.[2] There is a focus on love and belonging needs in addition to an emphasis on satisfying esteem needs.

The occupational therapist is interested in the influence of unresolved complexes upon the ability to satisfy these higher level needs. Concern for maintaining personal causation in a stressful environment is incorporated into the treatment approach. Additionally, the process of self-actualization is implemented in order that the substance abuser begins experiencing sobriety as potentially rewarding and satisfying.

Personal Causation

According to Kielhofner, personal causation is defined as a "collection of beliefs and expectations which a person holds about his or her effectiveness in the environment."[1] Personal causation involves attitudes regarding internal versus external control, belief in skills, belief in efficacy of skills and expectancy of success versus failure. A healthy sense of personal causation is evidenced by a person who believes in ability to be in control through the effective and successful use of skills.

Personal causation is addressed by emphasizing confidence in abilities regardless of emerging barriers to performance. Strategies to remove barriers are therefore an important factor in treatment at this level. For example, many substance abusers, after leaving inpatient or intensive outpatient treatment, often experience what is referred to as a "treatment high." Sobriety feels good, especially in the wake of the personal attention and understanding received from family, fellow substance abusers and staff of the treatment facility. The substance abuser feels confident and perhaps has overestimated personal efficacy in terms of ability to handle all possible stressful situations. Eventually, reality takes hold and the substance abuser's personal causation is badly shaken. Problems that may have been minimized while in treatment have not gone away and in some instances have grown in seriousness.

The goal of treatment level three is to shore up this badly damaged sense of personal causation. The therapist ensures that all the coping strategies taught during treatment level two are mobilized so that barriers to performance can be removed or at least modified. In some instances, acceptance of the problem is the only choice. Monitoring the impact of this now shaky sense of efficacy upon interests, values and goals is important. Lack of confidence, for example, could reduce willingness to explore new interests. Goals may be abandoned prematurely due to lack of belief in ability to succeed. Valuing sobriety eventually is undermined when no longer viewing abstinence as capable of producing satisfaction and enjoyment.

Self-Awareness

Expression of unconscious emotions produces an increase in self-awareness.[2] Without an adequate understanding of the self, self-concept is often impaired. Self-awareness occurs when the substance abuser verbalizes the complexes that trigger strong affect. Negative affect (depressed mood, fear, guilt, shame, anxiety, etc.) associated with symbol production provides cues regarding the existence of unresolved complexes.[2] Emotionality produced in connection with symbols alerts the therapist that deep-seated issues are governing behavior. The therapist facilitates recognition of negative affect and encourages further exploration to discern the extent of the complex(es). For substance abusers, the typical complexes are understanding reality, trust, intimacy, adequacy, dependence/independence, sexuality, aggression and loss.[10]

Projective techniques are utilized to facilitate production of symbols by the substance abuser that indicate the nature of the complex. Mosey states that symbols are best understood by considering their representation, form, and content.[2] Representation refers to "the way in which a symbol is produced," eg. exocepts (actions), images, endocepts (feelings), concepts or concrete objects.[2] Form of the symbol involves the "manifest structure" and might be exhibited, for example, as an animal or inanimate object.[2] Content includes the personal, cultural or archetypic meaning attributed to the symbol. Archetypic symbols refer to universal questions related to the suffering of human beings.[2] Cultural symbols involve values, norms and concerns of a particular culture, whereas idiosyncratic (personal) symbols reflect the unique experience of the individual.

The occupational therapist offers tentative interpretation of these symbols, facilitating insight into the complexes. The substance abuser verbalizes the meaning of the symbol, and by doing so, is scrutinizing the unconscious material through secondary process organization (logical thought).[2] Through logical analysis of this unconscious material, the substance abuser determines needs that are not being met. The substance abuser uses this self-knowledge to initiate behaviors that will lead to satisfaction of unresolved needs. The necessary energy to invest in appropriate need satisfaction is now available as the result of freeing complexes from the unconscious.

The occupational therapist suggests specific tasks and activities that assist the substance abuser in obtaining identified needs and resolving typical complexes. Mosey proposes that concerns about reality are resolved through participation in activities that include an evaluative component.[10] These activities encourage the substance abuser to make judgments regarding the environment and the self in the environment.

Trust issues are dealt with by activities that require sharing and cooperation in order to succeed.[10] Interaction with others contributes to satisfying needs for intimacy. Adequacy conflicts can be dealt with by successful completion of activities according to specified standards. Graded activities of increasing independence are designed for substance abusers with issues of dependency. Along with involvement in mixed sex groups, a supportive climate is necessary to enhance acceptance of sexuality. Developing assertive skills resolves conflicts of aggression. Sharing feelings related to loss decrease the negative influence upon function created by these unconscious concerns.

Insight into unconscious feelings is useless unless it is accompanied by development of mastery and control over these feelings. Without development of control, the substance abuser may avoid further projective experiences. There is a strong fear that feelings could totally overwhelm and consume the substance abuser. Losing control over emotions contributes to the relapse/inefficacy cycle.[11] The occupational therapist determines the substance abuser's ability to "integrate new insight into awareness and put it into action."[12] Therefore, even though insight is the goal of treatment, constructively acting on insight is evidence of ability to adaptively cope with all types of circumstances.

Self-Actualization

Self-actualization is defined by Mosey as "discovery of one's assets, limitations, and potentials."[10] Knowledge of the self leads to self-acceptance and understanding of one's place in time and space. Validation from others or approval seeking are not motivators for performance. Treatment is implied in the definition of self-actualization. The substance abuser engages in treatment activities that facilitate exploration of assets, limitations and potentials.

Self-actualization attaches meaning to a sober lifestyle. According to Frankl, continued feelings of meaninglessness can lead to addiction as well as aggression and depression.[13] Based on Frankl's theory, Crumbaugh developed logoanalysis therapy.[14,15] Crumbaugh and Carr demonstrated that logoanalysis improved sense of life meaning.[16] Hutzell replicated Crumbaugh's findings and demonstrated that logoanlysis group members versus control group members consistently exhibited more behavior changes indicative of positive attitudes toward a drug-independent life.[17]

This is not to say that the occupational therapist should implement logoanalysis programs. Emphasizing life meaning that can be generated from sobriety is crucial. Recall that many substance abusers relapse as a result of memories of positive affect experienced when using drugs.[11] Sobriety has to compete with these memories of positive affect and often fails. The substance abuser has difficulty finding meaning in ordinary routines. Activities that promote discovery of unused potentials and facilitate use of these new abilities are important.

In promoting self-actualization, the occupational therapist recognizes the substance abuser's self-actualizing behaviors when they occur. The occupational therapist points out these behaviors to the substance abuser in order to create awareness that desired growth is happening. According to Small, five classes of behaviors indicate that self-actualization is in process.[9] These five behaviors include experiencing the moment more fully and vividly, choosing a growth experience over an avoidance experience, checking out the belief system, engaging in arduous preparation for a chosen task, and recounting an increase in "peak experiences."

For example, self-actualization is proceeding when the substance abuser chooses a painful growth experience, such as admitting the extent of drug use, instead of lying or covering up. Challenging familiar methods of interpreting or perceiving events is another indication of self-actualization. Certain habits or behavior patterns may be questioned as to their importance or relevance. Self-actualization is in process when growth experiences are actively solicited, as is the case when deciding to go back to school.

Values Dysfunction

Values dysfunction is addressed by resolving conflicts within the existing value structure. Typical conflicts represent the contrast in beliefs previously held towards drugs and the new ideas regarding sobriety. Developing insight into the values conflict and acting on this insight is an important treatment emphasis. Treatment additionally focuses upon the effect of the value system in pursuing goals. Occupational performances in new roles depends upon selecting activities consistent with valued interests.

Values Conflicts

Values play a role in the development of unconscious conflicts. Values and social norms contributed to the substance abuser's beliefs and perceptions regarding drugs prior to the onset of chronic drug use.[18] During treatment level one, the substance abuser learned to value sobriety and during treatment level two, the substance abuser learned to value adaptive coping behaviors. Treatment level three requires investigation of conflicts within the value structure. Additionally, it is important that the substance abuser use the value system as a guide in selecting adaptive behaviors. Relying on a value system to guide behavior and to influence choices is a mark of a self-actualizing individual.

Conflicts within the value system are expressed symbolically through subtle references to guilt and shame.[2] Symbols may indicate aggression being turned in toward the self and there may be avoidance of relationships that possess judgmental qualities. Another clue, indicating values conflict, is an excessive preoccupation with religion. Sometimes substance abusers become over-involved in the spiritual aspects of AA in lieu of developing other, just as important, occupational performance areas.

As was true of the self-awareness process, the substance abuser engages in activities that promote projection of this values conflict. The values conflict is often expressed through the process of transference. Transference is defined by Mosey "as an unconscious psychological process characterized by a response to a person in a manner similar to the way in which one responded to a significant individual in one's past life."[10] The therapist may be viewed as similar to a person in the substance abuser's past that was particularly critical of the substance abuser's abilities. From this level of symbolic expression, the values conflict is brought to the verbal or conscious level.

Insight allows the substance abuser to evaluate whether the nature of the values conflict is such that change is required. If change is considered necessary, the "working through" process is begun.[10] Working through requires the substance abuser to come face-to-face with situations that invoke the values complex. Instead of continuing to act as was typical of the past, the substance abuser produces more adaptive behaviors. When the substance abuser discovers the fallacy of the ingrained beliefs, the strength of the complex is greatly reduced.

Valued Goals

An important part of personal causation, especially in terms of persistence in effort, is the individual's value system.[1] Being able to pursue a goal over a length of time and to continue the effort regardless of barriers to performance depends upon internalized values. A person who values career advancement, for example, will spend more time engaged in these pursuits versus an individual who values time spent with family members. Achievement requires that values be identified so that corresponding effort can be mobilized to accomplish the related goals. Confusing values create goal conflicts that interfere with achievement.

During this treatment level, the substance abuser may experience a challenge to the recently acquired value of sobriety. Perhaps a strong desire for socialization wins precedence over sobriety. Because of feeling more comfortable during socialization activities when drinking or using drugs, there is temptation to revert to the old methods of coping. In this situation, the valued socialization erodes the value of sobriety.

For instance, a female substance abuser comes to group stating that with the advent of sobriety, she never has fun anymore. Group members confront the substance abuser regarding the possibility that having fun at any cost is more important than sobriety. Also the group encourages the substance abuser to define her concept of fun, uncovering that fun is not the value in operation. The real value taking precedence over sobriety relates to the feelings generated by alcohol and other drugs, ie. increased sense of power, sexuality and loss of inhibition. The substance abuser is helped to identify other activities that could produce the same emotions, eg. the sense of power resulting from deliberate and successful engagement in a desired task. In this way, the values clash is redefined and the substance abuser can direct goal pursuit in more fruitful directions.

Expanded Roles

Taking on new roles is an important aspect of achievement. As a result of self-development and calculated risk taking, the substance abuser is ready to take on new roles that previously were never seriously considered. Treatment level two focused upon developing skills necessary for routine role performance. By contrast, treatment level three prepares the substance abuser for new roles. Skill exploration and skill practice ensure development of competence. The occupational therapist helps the substance abuser realize the relationship between sobriety and ability to engage in these expanded role opportunities.

Reactions to these new roles are explored, especially in light of heightened self-awareness and knowledge of personal values. Strong negative responses to new role situations are brought to the substance abuser's attention, with resulting encouragement to explore this possibly symbolic behavior. Exploring reactions to new roles is important for substance abusers who use alcohol and drugs as a self-handicapping strategy.[19] Use of drugs may ensure that the substance abuser does not have to be responsible when failing. Positive self-image is dependent upon past successful performances and not on current or future performances. Because of fear of failure, the substance abuser is not interested in trying out new, risky behaviors or roles, especially now that drugs are not available to hide incompetency.[19]

Insight is developed by determining the influence of fear of failure and the need for self-handicapping strategies. The substance abuser determines if this adequacy complex interferes with current occupational behavior. Given that the substance abuser is willing to make changes, the therapist facilitates the working-through process.

◆ OCCUPATIONAL THERAPY GROUPS ◆

At treatment level three, groups are designed that confront continued use of maladaptive defense mechanisms and promote insight into the issues related to addiction. Groups are confrontational in nature, thereby forcing the substance abuser to use previously learned adaptive coping strategies. Three types of occupational therapy groups are utilized to accomplish the objective of enhancing personal growth. These three types include task-oriented groups, developmental groups, and instrumental groups.

The two developmental groups are cooperative groups and mature groups (Table 7-3). Task-oriented groups are defined by Mosey as helping members become "aware of their needs, values, ideas, and feelings as they influence action, and to test the validity of this intrapsychic content".[10] Instrumental groups maintain function and do not instigate change.[10]

At treatment level three, group members are usually outpatients. Group content focuses on psychological performance components, especially issues related to self-concept. Occupational performances developed through work and leisure activities continue to be important at this treatment level. However, groups involve more complex skills training and the refinement of previously learned skills. Direct experience with the expected environment is reported back to the outpatient occupational therapy groups to monitor successes and assist with problem-solving.

TASK-ORIENTED GROUPS

Skill in group interaction is not the focus of this group format, although it may occur secondarily. The primary goal of the task-oriented group is self-awareness or self-understanding.[10] Activities elicit behavior which can be explored. Group members analyze the thoughts and feelings that promoted a specific behavioral reaction.

Table 7-3
Treatment Level Three Groups

Group	Factors to be Considered with Substance Abusers	Strategies
Cooperative Group	Ability to interact in homogeneous groups Ability to express feelings, and perceive and meet needs of others	Meal preparation Leisure planning Group craft projects
Mature Group	Involvement in intense relationships Ability to cooperate	Group work tasks Volunteer committee work
Task Group	Readiness to develop self-awareness or self-understanding	Projective activities Group processing
Instrumental Group	Maintenance of new skills requiring satisfaction of current needs	Level two thematic groups Assertiveness training Anger management

Tasks are selected by group members that facilitate discussion of pertinent issues. During the actual task completion, the substance abuser experiences the influence of personal values, thoughts and feelings on actions, on relationships with others, and on the completion of the task. For example, a task involving intensive physical activity may indicate unresolved issues related to hostility and aggression.

During the initial stages of the group, discussion typically centers around the task itself. This concrete discussion gives group members a basic grounding in reality before proceeding to more abstract levels of behavioral insight. As trust develops between group members, the discussion usually turns to interpersonal relations. Slowly the group members feel comfortable in sharing negative and positive feelings about themselves. Discussions conducted after task engagement, encourage awareness of behavior, stimulate insight into causes of behavior, and identify methods of altering unacceptable behaviors and resolving negative feelings.

Task-oriented groups incorporate the principles of insight development and the working through process. The therapist's leadership role varies depending on the trust levels between group members, insight and verbal ability of group members. Group members assume responsibilities as co-therapists relative to other group members. Group members learn that they are an essential part in helping each other.

The occupational therapist utilizes the task-oriented group to confront continued usage of maladaptive defense mechanisms. The group members are cautioned to look out for these behaviors in each other. The group is particularly sensitive to behaviors indicative of denial, projection, rationalization, dichotomies, the avoiding or minimization of conflicts, obsessiveness or selective self-centered attention. When any of these maladaptive behavioral strategies occur, the substance abuser is confronted and is encouraged to examine the stress that may have contributed to PDS use. The substance abuser is then assisted in implementing learned coping strategies, such as assertive communication, anger management or cognitive restructuring.

For instance, consider that the task-oriented group chose to make collages illustrating the meaning of sobriety. Perhaps one group member is not working and when confronted, denies that this is true by rationalizing about being tired. The other group members point out that this pattern of behavior has been exhibited consistently during several group sessions. The confronted substance abuser responds to the criticism by overworking for the next half-hour of the group session and even though angry, fails to express the feelings except through nonverbal behaviors. The angry substance abuser eventually begins to snap at several of the group members.

Finally, an insightful group member points out to the substance abuser and the rest of the group members the series of PDS behaviors exhibited, ie. denial, rationalization, dichotomous behavior, conflict avoidance and displacement. The angry substance abuser is assisted in exploring his reluctance to participate and to share these feelings honestly with the group. "I have had strong urges to use lately. I've been under stress at work to complete a project I don't feel capable of handling. I bought a bottle of liquor and hid it in the garage." Problem-solving is instituted during group sessions. With the help of a selected group member, the substance abuser phones his AA sponsor to meet him at home after group in order to remove the bottle of alcohol. The rest of the group session then focuses on methods to handle stress and improve feelings of personal causation.

The task-oriented group is a powerful treatment tool available to occupational therapists. The group serves to integrate the coping skills acquired from the other two treatment levels. Through this type of group interaction, the substance abuser is cognizant of maladaptive coping produced from stressful situations and responds by altering inappropriate behaviors with newly learned skills and strategies. The group serves as a laboratory where it is acceptable to make mistakes and try out new learning. Problems experienced after making the decision to commit to abstinence surface during these groups. The group member benefits from the help and understanding of fellow group members. Relapse is thus prevented by the offering of support in times of stress. Stress can threaten belief in ability to cope other than through the consumption of alcohol and other drugs.

COOPERATIVE GROUPS

Cooperative groups are similar to egocentric-cooperative groups except for their homogeneous membership.[10] Homogeneity may occur on a variety of factors in addition to the usual "male" restricted or "female" restricted group. The fact that all the group members are substance abusers contributes to the homogeneity. The occupational therapist may select group members based on drug of choice and personality type, ie. using drugs for activation, relaxation or escape into fantasy.

It is advantageous to conduct a group exclusive for female substance abusers. The literature indicates that there are differences between male and female substance abusers. In terms of alcoholism, these differences include the fact that women: 1) typically consume less alcohol than men, 2) begin both drinking and problem drinking at a later age, 3) progress more rapidly to chronic alcoholism ("telescoping"), 4) attribute onset to specific life stress, 5) experience more stigma than men because of drinking, 6) have affective disorders, 7) experience the consequences of drinking in terms of family disruption, 8) have an alcoholic role model in the nuclear family, 9) demonstrate different medical sequelae, and 10) feel guilty, anxious, or depressed.[20,21]

In a cooperative group, the task is secondary to the group process.[10] There is more opportunity than there was in the egocentric-cooperative group to express both positive and negative feelings, to perceive the needs of others and to meet the needs of others. The egocentric-cooperative level two group focused exclusively on self-esteem needs; whereas, the level three cooperative group addresses a variety of need satisfaction issues. The cooperative group is differentiated from the task-oriented group by its focus on group interaction skill. This is not the purpose of the task-oriented group, which emphasizes examination of intrapsychic content.

The cooperative group is an excellent outpatient group format as it serves three basic purposes: 1) supplies warmth and cohesion that resembles family solidarity, 2) provides opportunities to experiment with social adaptation such as love, cooperation and disagreement, and 3) allows experience of giving to others as well as receiving.[10] The therapist's role in this group varies, but primarily, the occupational therapist retains a low profile. Initially, the therapist ensures that the group develops a strong sense of cohesiveness, identity and specialness. Cohesiveness is fostered by maintaining adequate frequency of interaction, selecting group members with definite similarities, creating expectations for successful experiences and maintaining a climate conducive to cooperation and democratic leadership.

During the formative group stages, the therapist may be participating in a manner similar to other group members by freely sharing feelings and ideas. Authoritarian attitudes are avoided. Without this emotional aspect of cohesiveness, the group members may not be able to express positive or negative emotions and ideas.[10] Eventually, as the group matures, the therapist withdraws from active daily participation and begins to fulfill the roles of providing external support and consultation.

Because of the need for cohesiveness and specialness, the group is time limited and closed. Movement of new members in and out of the group defeats these purposes. Tasks selected by the group members emphasize enjoyment, sharing and avoid complexity so that the task does not overshadow group interaction. Spectator activities are not encouraged as there are few opportunities for interaction.[10] The creative arts such as poetry, dancing, listening to music and completing art work offer rich opportunities for the cooperative group. The format of the group typically alternates between doing an activity and talking about feelings and ideas aroused by the activity. However, the purpose of the group is not to discuss intrapsychic content. As Mosey states, "there is no attempt to develop in-depth self-understanding or to alter feelings and ideas. The purpose of the group is simply to be able to share on an emotional level."[10]

Group members develop strong friendships. In fact, the substance abuser pursues cooperative group memberships in the community in order to retain interactions that satisfy a variety of personal needs. These memberships, as stated in regard to the egocentric-cooperative group, are vital in avoiding relapse. The cooperative group provides sources of positive affect divorced from drug use that increase the attractiveness of sobriety to the recovering substance abuser.

MATURE GROUPS

The mature group develops group interaction skills that balance task oriented and social maintenance behaviors.[10] This group skill is necessary for successful occupational performance required by the individual's job or volunteer activities. The substance abuser learns to work with others in order to get the job done, but also learns to promote and foster working relationships. Presented in this manner, the substance abuser understands the necessity of learning instrumental and expressive group roles.

Instrumental roles are those functions necessary for task completion and often include: 1) the initiator-contributor or the individual who suggests new ideas, 2) the information seeker or the one who asks for clarification of facts, 3) the opinion seeker or the one who asks for clarification of opinions or values, 4) the information giver or the one who offers facts, 5) the elaborator or the one who expounds on suggestions, 6) the coordinator or the clarifier of relationships, 7) the orienter or the one who defines the position of the group with respect to its goals, 8) the evaluator critic or the one who compares group accomplishments to standards, and 9) the procedural technician or the one who expedites task performance.[10]

Expressive roles gratify the needs of group members and monitor the social function of the group as a whole. These expressive roles include: 1) the encourager or the one who praises, agrees with, and accepts the contributions of others, 2) the harmonizer or the one who mediates differences between group members, 3) the compromiser or the one who changes behavior to maintain harmony, 4) the gatekeeper or the one who facilitates and maintains communication, 5) the standard setter or the one who expresses the standards set by the group, 6) the group observer or the one who notes, interprets and gives information regarding the group process, and 7) the follower or the one who goes along with the movement of the group.[10]

Group members take turns observing group interactions as a method of learning these various group roles. The group can momentarily suspend its work on tasks to examine the group roles exhibited and can even take time to role-play new roles that members are having difficulty assuming. The therapist, in the mature group, assumes the role of a peer. In fact, the group observer points out when the group members are becoming too dependent upon the therapist and when the therapist is subtly being coerced into a leadership role.

The mature group also considers taking time out from group interactions to share mature group experiences that occur during the normal daily routine. This is an important method of enhancing transfer of training and increases the relevancy of the group. In this way, the substance abuser applies the group roles learned in therapy to real-life situations, especially those interactions occurring on the job. Stressful group experiences that happen at work are shared with the mature group in order to determine group role strategies available to the substance abuser.

INSTRUMENTAL GROUPS

This group does not make behavioral changes, but maintains functioning levels already obtained or that are in danger of being lost.[10] With this definition, it seems that the group purpose is not congruent with the insight development goal of treatment level three. There is an additional function relegated to aftercare programs. That purpose concerns the transfer and maintenance of previously learned skills to the real environment.

After discharge from an inpatient treatment setting or a reduction in intensive outpatient programming, a goal of aftercare is the maintenance of sobriety through supporting the substance abuser's newly learned coping mechanisms. As the substance abuser becomes more sure or believes more strongly in efficacy of coping, instrumental groups are discontinued. Instrumental groups are especially important for those substance abusers who are returning to or who are currently living in nonsupportive home environments. These substance abusers have high risks of relapse and are in danger of losing newly learned coping skills.

Instrumental groups are extensions of thematic groups conducted at treatment level two. The instrumental groups continue the emphasis on social skills, cognitive restructuring, problem-solving, anger management, stress reduction, lifestyle adjustment, time management, etc. The group gives supportive and constructive feedback to utilization of coping skills during real-life situations. Frustrations resulting from unrealistic expectations regarding the impact of effective coping are managed by the group. This group refocuses the substance abuser away from short-term gratification or expectation that immediate happiness should automatically result from coping appropriately. The instrumental group enhances realization that long-term changes will occur from maintained effective coping. Continued desire for immediate short-term gratification could lead to relapse and the belief that alcohol and drugs can immediately satisfy needs in a way that exceeds the effect of behavioral changes.

Instrumental groups prevent relapse and are used for relapsing substance abusers that do not require inpatient hospitalization. Actually, instrumental groups are employed at all treatment levels. These groups are necessary for those substance abusers who are unable to progress from one treatment level to another. This is particularly true for treatment level one substance abusers who fail to obtain adequate levels of cognitive recovery or treatment level two substance abusers who never develop the ego strength necessary for insight oriented approaches characteristic of treatment level three.

The goal of an instrumental group targeted for substance abusers with permanent cognitive deficits is to maximize existing cognitive functioning through adaptation of the environment and training of caregivers. For substance abusers with weak ego strength, the goal of the instrumental group is to maintain existing coping abilities, thereby fostering self-esteem and self-confidence. Eventually, the substance abuser may achieve the necessary ego strength that allows exploration of the issues of addiction.

◆ TREATMENT TERMINATION ◆

Termination of treatment does not occur abruptly, but involves a gradual process whenever possible. In time, termination becomes a topic between the therapist and the substance abuser. At the point where it appears that termination is imminent, the substance abuser and the occupational therapist formulate a phasing-out process. Mutual understanding that this phasing-out can change, if needed, will calm the substance abuser's fears. One method of phasing out is to gradually reduce the frequency of the treatment sessions and group participation. The door to treatment remains open if the substance abuser needs reassurance from time to time. It is made clear that the substance abuser is expected to continue involvement in AA/NA or other support groups, and that this support compliments the substance abuser's new found abilities.

The occupational therapist is aware of the stress related to pending treatment termination. Discharge from treatment often produces behaviors characteristic of older styles of coping. These "preparatory" behaviors are pointed out to the substance abuser so that reinstitution of more adaptive coping can take place. Sometimes these behaviors continue and create the need to postpone termination. In this situation, the substance abuser is symbolically indicating that termination plans are premature.

◆ REEVALUATION ◆

Another concern regarding termination is the failure to discontinue treatment in a timely manner. Continuing treatment beyond the point of making significant gains in function could facilitate dependency upon the therapist, group members or the treatment system. Many substance abusers display dependency issues throughout treatment. Some substance abusers with severe dependency issues have to be weaned from therapy as soon as possible. This means that the occupational therapist discerns, through reevaluation, differences between typical behaviors triggered by threat of termination and behaviors that indicate need for continued treatment.

As was true of the other treatment levels, reevaluation focuses upon long- and short-term goal accomplishment. Pre- and post-measuring are important to establish improvements in baseline functioning. Improvements are noted in self-concept, self-actualization, identification of values, utilization of values to make decisions and skills necessary for expanded roles.

Treatment termination is postponed when reevaluation indicates lack of progress. Lack of progress necessitates revision in treatment approaches or in the treatment goals. Poor results could indicate premature advancement to treatment level three. In this case, instrumental groups that emphasize treatment level two skills are important.

◆ CONCLUSIONS ◆

This chapter identified frames of reference capable of developing insight and confronting continued reliance upon the PDS. Object relations and model of human occupation both stimulate personality growth. Object relations is the most adept at facilitating insight compared to the model of human occupation which emphasizes role and values development.

Functional evaluation determines the influence of psychological factors of self-awareness, personal causation and self-actualization upon expanded role performance. Values dysfunction also inhibits functional performance. Treatment planning reflects diagnosed occupational role and performance dysfunctions along with the underlying contributors to these problems. Treatment strategies involve insight development through activities that promote symbol production. Symbols are analyzed at the conscious level. The substance abuser determines need to change, institutes active coping and begins the working through process. Strength of the unconscious complex is thereby reduced.

Treatment level three groups confront any existing reliance on the PDS and foster insight development through exploration of the issues of addiction. Cooperative, mature, task-oriented, and instrumental groups are characteristic of the groups designed for treatment level three. Reevaluation determines need for treatment termination. Termination involves a phasing out process. Reverting to maladaptive coping strategies often occurs during termination and requires confrontation. Occasionally, the substance abuser is symbolically indicating need for further treatment. It is necessary to distinguish between the legitimate need for continued treatment and expression of routine fears. The risk is to prolong treatment unnecessarily, thereby promoting continued dependence upon the treatment system.

References

1. Kielhofner G (Ed): *A Model of Human Occupation: Theory and Application.* Baltimore, MD: Williams and Wilkins, 1985, pp. 64, 70, 15.
2. Mosey AC: *Three Frames of Reference for Mental Health.* Thorofare, NJ: Slack Inc., 1970.
3. Maslow A: *Toward a Psychology of Being.* Princeton, NJ: D. Van Nostrand Company, Inc., 1962.
4. Wallace J: Behavioral modification methods as adjuncts to psychotherapy. In Zimberg S, Wallace J, Blume SB (Eds.): *Practical Approaches to Alcoholism Psychotherapy* (2nd ed.). New York: Plenum Press, 1985.
5. Pattison EM: Types of alcoholism reflective of character disorders. In Zales M (Ed.): *Character Pathology.* New York: Bruner/Mazel, 1983.
6. Shostrom EL: *Personal Orientation Inventory (POI) Manual.* San Diego, CA: EDITS, 1966 & 1974.
7. Hutzell RR, Peterson TJ: Use of the life purpose questionnaire with an alcoholic population. *Int J Addict* 21(1): 51-57, 1986.
8. Quereshi MY: The development of the Michill Adjective Rating Scale (MARS). *J Clin Psychol* 26: 192-196, 1970.
9. Small JS: *Becoming Naturally Therapeutic.* Austin, TX: The Eupsychian Press, 1981, pp. 59, 67, 72, 52, 53.
10. Mosey AC: *Psychosocial Components of Occupational Therapy.* New York: Raven Press, 1986, pp. 39, 398, 280, 287, 252.
11. Marlatt GA, Gordon JR: *Relapse Prevention.* New York: Guilford Press, 1985.
12. Bruce MA, Borg B: *Frames of Reference in Psychosocial Occupational Therapy.* Thorofare, NJ: Slack Inc., 1987.
13. Frankl VE: *The Will to Meaning: Foundations and Applications of Logotherapy.* New York: World Publishing, 1969.
14. Crumbaugh JC: *Everything to Gain. A Guide to Self-fulfillment Through Logoanalysis.* Chicago: Nelson Hall, 1973.

15. Crumbaugh JC, Wood WM, Wood WC: *Logotherapy: New Help for Problem Drinkers*. Chicago: Nelson Hall, 1980.

16. Crumbaugh JC, Carr GL: Treatment of alcoholics with logotherapy. *Int J Addict* 14(6): 847-853, 1979.

17. Hutzell RR: Logoanalysis for alcoholics. *Int For Logother* 7: 40-45, 1984.

18. Biddle BJ, Bank BJ, Marlin MM: Social determinants of adolescent drinking: What they think, what they do and what I think they do. *J Stud Alcohol* 41: 215-241, 1980.

19. Hull JG, Young RD: Self-consciousness, self-esteem, and success-failure as determinants of alcohol consumption in male social drinkers. *J Pers Soc Psychol* 44: 1097-1109, 1983.

20. Blume S: Clinical research: Casefinding, diagnosis, treatment, and rehabilitation. In *Alcohol and Women*. (Research Monograph no. 1). Rockville, MD: National Institute on Alcohol Abuse and Alcoholism, 1980, pp. 121-149.

21. Braiker HB: The diagnosis and treatment of alcoholism in women. *Special Population Issues*. (Alcohol and Health Monograph no. 4). Rockville, MD: National Institute on Alcohol Abuse and Alcoholism, 1982, pp. 111-139.

Family Treatment
and Occupational Therapy

INTRODUCTION

Substance abuse is a family problem. Focusing exclusively in therapy on the addicted individual causes one to lose sight of the "big picture." Individual treatment of the substance abuser is at best a partial treatment. Even though it is generally understood that substance abuse affects the entire family, occupational therapists tend to approach treatment in isolation of the family structure. This is true of occupational therapy partly because of the fairly recent inclusion of family approaches as an aspect of substance abuse treatment. However, now that intervention normally includes a family component, occupational therapy has been slow to establish a role in this treatment area.

The literature does delineate an occupational therapy intervention approach, further described in this chapter, for treating the family impacted by substance abuse.[1-3] The occupational therapy literature in general, though, is just beginning to address the influence of the family upon an individual's occupational performance. For example, issues of the family are appearing in terms of parent-child relationships of handicapped children and in terms of caregiving provided for the elderly.[4-9]

There is an emerging emphasis in occupational therapy upon family treatment in promoting recovery from substance abuse and from occupational dysfunction. This chapter describes the occupational therapy family treatment approach that is distinct from methods utilized by other professionals. The family treatment approach closely corresponds to the substance abuser's occupational therapy program. The three hierarchical treatment levels match occupational therapy treatment for the family with the appropriate family system characteristics and stage of family recovery.

◆ THE FAMILY SYSTEM ◆

To further understand the devastating effects of substance abuse upon the entire family, the family can be viewed as a system.[10] A family system is made up of individual members or system components that assume specific roles. These roles dictate the interaction between family members. Family relationships conducted according to the rules of the system maintain the family equilibrium.[11] Given shifts in the family equilibrium, such as substance abuse, the entire family must adapt to the painful stress. Often the strategies individual family members use to adapt to stress produce temporary results and create more problems then they solve.[12]

Wegscheider describes the major rules often associated with alcoholic family systems.[13] The family functioning is guided by the belief that the individual's substance abuse is the most important aspect of family life. However, drugs are not considered the cause of the family's problems. Someone or something else is believed to perpetuate the substance abuse. The person suffering from addiction is therefore not held responsible. The status quo must be maintained and family members diligently cover up for the individual's drug related indiscretions. No one may discuss what is really happening nor share true feelings.

◆ MALADAPTIVE FAMILY ROLES ◆

The substance abuser's preferred defense structure (PDS) profoundly influences the family system. Family members unfortunately do not recognize the substance abuser's dependence upon maladaptive defense mechanisms. A common mistake is for the family to expect rational reactions when the substance abuser encounters stress or conflict. This lack of understanding by the family could actually perpetuate the substance abuser's drug use.

The entire family system eventually becomes caught up in the problem of substance abuse. Wegscheider describes six family roles and these include the chemically dependent person, the chief enabler, the family hero, the scapegoat, the lost child and the mascot.[13] Each family role hides feelings and contributes a valuable function to the family.[13] For example, the chief enabler, often the spouse, is overly responsible and increasingly assumes the duties vacated by the substance abuser. The family hero, through efforts of achievement, brings a sense of pride to the family, while simultaneously covering up the family's fear of failure. The scapegoat's angry, defiant behavior removes the family's focus from substance abuse so that denial of parental addiction may continue. The scapegoat expresses for the entire family the anger and rage engendered by the substance abuser.

Withdrawal and isolation of the lost child brings relief to the family.[13] The family believes that the lost child is not in need of energy from the rest of the system, thus available energy is conserved for "more important concerns." The lost child demonstrates the family's sense of powerlessness and helplessness. The mascot, like the lost child, also gives relief to the family, but this relief is in the form of tension release. The clowning and joking behavior masks underlying emotions of terror and hysteria.

Actually, these roles are not discrete categories. Family members assume a blend of these roles. The role combinations of a family member fluctuate as a result of changes in the system.[13] For instance, if the scapegoat's problematic behavior is resolved, possibly as the result of therapeutic intervention, another family member may be forced to take over this now vacant role. Treatment for the substance abuser requires that total confrontation be delayed until the PDS can be replaced with alternative, more healthy coping strategies and defense mechanisms. This same principal of careful confrontation is applied to family members. Family members cannot relinquish their maladaptive roles unless other, more adaptive behaviors are learned in response to the positive changes in the substance abuser's behavior. The family needs to understand the influence of the substance abuser's PDS during addiction, treatment and recovery.

Treatment of substance abusers thus includes the resolution of family system issues. If change occurs in the substance abuser and not in the family, the family system may respond with homeostatic transactions that promote addictive behaviors. Additionally, the family may actually sabotage continued treatment in order to maintain the system's balance. Jacob and Leonard state that addiction has adaptive consequences for the family, which can reinforce and perpetuate patterns of abusive drug use.[14]

◆ PDS VARIABLES ◆

The family displays specific PDS variables that impact treatment outcomes. These characteristics were previously described for the substance abuser as needing external control at treatment level one, internal control at treatment level two, and insight at treatment level three. The family's therapeutic issues also correspond with a particular treatment level. These issues include relinquishing maladaptive role behavior at treatment level one, developing coping behaviors at treatment level two, and stimulating growth at treatment level three (Table 8-1).

As with the substance abuser, these issues are operationally defined in terms of the family's strengths and weaknesses (Table 8-2). In terms of treatment level one, if the family reports enabling the addiction, the family corrects these styles of interacting in order to augment the external control needed by the substance abuser. Such behaviors as emptying the substance abuser's liquor bottles or destroying the drug supply, putting the substance abuser to bed when intoxicated, bailing the substance abuser out of jail, and calling work to state the substance abuser is sick are all forms of enabling that remove responsibility from the substance abuser.

Currently, the term "co-dependent" signifies the nonaddicted family members or significant others (eg. employers, coworkers or friends) whose health and behavior not only influence the person suffering from addiction, but who are also negatively affected by the same individual.[15] Children or adult co-dependents may display such psychiatric symptoms as anxiety, depression, insomnia, hyperactivity, aggression, anorexia nervosa, bulimia and suicidal gestures.[16] Family violence, child neglect or chemical dependency in other family members may also result.[17]

Therefore, at treatment level one, family enabling is replaced by healthy methods of responding to the substance abuser's drug habits. The family learns to provide external control which assists the substance abuser to obtain sobriety. External control differs from enabling. The family creates expectations for responsible behavior and administers consequences for the inappropriate behaviors displayed by the substance abuser.

With progression to treatment level two, the family has stopped enabling. They probably have difficulty coping with the daily stresses of life. For too long, family members have been

Table 8-1
Substance Abuser and Family Characteristics Impacting Treatment Matching

	PDS Variables (Characteristics)	
Treatment Level	Family Role Changes	Substance Abuser PDS
1	Relinquish enabling	External control
2	Develop coping	Internal control
3	Stimulate growing	Insight

Table 8-2
PDS Variables Operationalized

	Operationalized PDS Variables	
Treatment Level	Substance Abuser PDS	Family Role Changes
1	Loss of control over substance use	Enabler, Victim, Adjuster, Hero, Mascot, Scapegoat, Lost Child
2	Difficulty coping with daily problems/needing assistance to stay sober	Difficulty coping with personal issues
3	Responding to unresolved conflicts	Trapped in growth curtailing roles Lack of insight

preoccupied with the substance abuser's drug use. They typically have ignored personal needs. A variety of healthy coping strategies are learned and incorporated by the family into daily routines during treatment level two. With the advent of treatment level three, the family is coping adequately. Now, the family explores the dynamics of the family environment that promoted addictive behavior.

◆ TREATMENT VARIABLES ◆

PDS STATUS

Recall that treatment variables involve the concepts of PDS status, treatment methods and frame of reference (Tables 8-3 and 8-4). PDS status incorporates the three treatment levels. The levels correspond to changes in the substance abuser's preferred defense structure and the family's relinquishing of maladaptive roles. The family's role status does not remain static, but is changing as the result of treatment. The three treatment levels, outlined in Table 8-1, facilitate occupational therapy treatment matching decisions for the family. The relationship between the

Table 8–3
Treatment Variables Impacting Matching

Treatment Level	Substance Abuser's PDS Status	Family Role Status	Treatment Method
1	Mobilized	Relinquished	Directive
2	Weakened	Decentralized addiction	Supportive
3	Confronted	Gained insight	Confrontive

Table 8–4
Family Treatment Variables

Treatment Level	Family Role Status	Treatment Method	Frame of Reference
1	Relinquished	Directive	Action Consequence Model of Human Occupation Systems Theory
2	Decentralized addiction	Supportive	Cognitive-Behavioral Model of Human Occupation Systems Theory
3	Gained insight	Confrontive	Object Relationships Model of Human Occupation Systems Theory

substance abuser's PDS changes and the family's shifts from acting maladaptive roles to incorporating adaptive roles is illustrated.

During treatment level one, the substance abuser's PDS is mobilized and the family relinquishes such maladaptive roles as enabling or assuming a victim stance. At treatment level two, the substance abuser's PDS is weakened and the family members give importance to themselves, thus decentralizing addiction from the system. Finally, the substance abuser's PDS is thoroughly confronted by completion of level three. The family gains insight regarding its role in perpetuating addictive behavior.

TREATMENT METHODS

Treatment variables also include the type of treatment methods that produce change in the PDS and the family's role behavior at each level (see Table 8-3). Directive treatment methods are necessary for producing the external control and the relinquished family roles required during treatment level one. Supportive methods are used during treatment level two to teach new coping strategies. Confrontational methods are indicated by treatment level three. This approach deters continued usage of maladaptive roles and defense mechanisms.

FRAMES OF REFERENCE

Selecting a frame of reference for treatment of the family is similar to the process delineated for the substance abuser. Screening determines the treatment level corresponding to the needs of the family and helps select the appropriate frame of reference. Data from chart reviews, interviews and performance measures are utilized.

Individual interviews are employed when it is not possible to conduct the family interview with all family members present. The purposes of the family or individual interviews are to assess each member's position or role within the family system, to gather data regarding perceived family problems, to ascertain motivation and expectations for treatment, to determine levels of family stress and current stressors, to give an overview of the treatment program, and to strengthen the family's commitment to treatment. Performance measures evaluate specific skills of individual family members or require the family to interact together. During this interaction, the occupational therapist observes the family system dynamics.

Before a frame of reference is selected, though, the occupational therapist determines whether the family program incorporates the entire family as a unit, addresses issues of specific individuals or focuses on subcomponents of the family system. Frame of reference selection is easiest when dealing with one family member at a time. In this case, the frames of reference utilized for the substance abuser at each level apply to individual family members, eg. action-consequence at treatment level one or cognitive-behavioral at treatment level two. When treating the family as a whole or when addressing issues of specific subgroups of the family, systems theory is helpful in guiding evaluation, treatment planning, intervention and progress determination.

Systems theory focuses evaluation and treatment upon the input, throughput, output and feedback aspects of the family system.[18] The throughput process involves the relationships between the family members and the resultant communication patterns that are typical of the system. The output of the system is the functional behaviors of the family.[19] The family unit relates to the outside environment in order to obtain the necessary input for the system and to process feedback. The family system is an open system and, when appropriately taking in energy from outside itself, enters an adaptive cycle of change. Family systems that are isolated from the environment have only their own energy available. Potential for adaptation is severely limited.[20]

According to systems theory, evaluation and treatment addresses the maladaptive cycle of the family. Family functioning is modified and relationships with the environment are enhanced. Renewed relationships with the environment provide new inputs into the system and increase responsiveness to feedback. The throughput process is changed by enhancing constructive communication patterns, redesigning coalitions and reinforcing appropriate boundaries between family members.[20] The occupational therapist designs treatment strategies that work each family member into adaptive roles that correct the structural skews caused by substance abuse.

FAMILY TREATMENT APPROACHES

Occupational therapy intervention directed toward the family corresponds with the treatment dynamics of the substance abuser. Decisions are made regarding whether the family is treated separately or jointly with the substance abuser. A combination of strategies is often useful. During those times when the family is treated separately from the substance abuser, it is best that different occupational therapists, when possible, be assigned to the family and to the substance abuser. This preserves allegiance to the primary client for each occupational therapist. Both therapists work together during the joint sessions. These recommendations are based upon ideal staffing that does not always exist.

The number of family members that the occupational therapist can treat is objectively examined. Decisions depend upon the size of the family, the age ranges and the services offered by the family treatment program. In terms of age, children under eight years old are often excluded from traditional family therapy programs. Occupational therapists use modalities that accommodate young children's difficulty in verbalizing problems.

Occupational therapy treatment strategies address particular problems identified for subsystem components of the family. For example, occupational therapy sessions could focus upon the spouses' relationships, the parents' interactions with their children, the children's ability to cede parental responsibilities assumed prematurely, or the children's interactions with each other. Table 8-5 examines the relationship between treatment levels and the need for separate or joint family treatment. This table also delineates the treatment focus and corresponding occupational therapy family treatment strategies.

Treatment Level One

During treatment level one, the substance abuser is seen separately from the family. The substance abuser is responding to external control that succeeds in mobilizing the PDS toward abstinence. The family members shift their role from enabling to providing consequences for drug-related behaviors. The goals of treatment for the family at treatment level one involve

Table 8-5
Occupational Therapy Family Goals and Strategies

Treatment Level	Goals	Strategies	Family Therapy Type
1	Stress reduction Identifying maladaptive roles Decreasing game playing External control training Attitude retraining	Learning techniques: teaching, modeling, coaching, rehearsal, transfer of training Relaxation techniques Alcohol/drug education Household routines Leisure and exercise Catharsis	Separate
2	Coping skill development Problem-solving skill development Skill generalization Independent skill usage	Cognitive techniques: cognitive restructuring, cognitive rehearsal, thought stopping, cognitive appraisal, problem-solving Learning techniques Assertiveness training Stress management Time management	Joint Separate
3	Development of insight Skill generalization Mature family relationships Reduction of value conflicts Identifying new family roles	Projective techniques Group processing Problem-solving Confrontation of maladaptive roles Values clarification Goal-setting/planning for the future Learning technique Cognitive techniques	Joint Separate

reducing stress, augmenting ability to provide external control, and changing negative attitudes held toward the substance abuser.

Stress Reduction

The first emphasis of family-oriented occupational therapy is to reduce stress. Stress reduction allows the family to actively participate in treatment in order to gain needed skills. Occupational therapy helps the family to covertly reframe problems in a way that denotes expectation for problem solution. For example, family members may believe that their situation is hopeless and therefore no attempt to solve problems is made. Through treatment, the family successfully reduces the stress in their lives, thereby learning that positive changes can occur in response to their own efforts.

Family members reduce anxiety by implementing relaxation techniques learned in occupational therapy. A household daily routine controls the chaos often characteristic of families impacted by substance abuse. Other stress reduction activities are experienced in occupational therapy including instituting a balanced diet, engaging in exercise and selecting meaningful leisure activities.

Relinquishing Maladaptive Roles

Once stress is reduced, the family relinquishes maladaptive roles in order to augment the external control needed by the substance abuser. Providing external control does not indicate that the family controls the substance abuser's behavior. This is not possible. External control occurs when the family behaves in a way that helps the substance abuser achieve abstinence. Even though external control is beneficial for the substance abuser, primarily the family members benefit. The family members no longer place their own feelings as subservient to the needs of the substance abuser. The family members help the substance abuser by helping themselves. The family administers consequences or lets the substance abuser suffer the effects of drug use, eg. getting fired or sleeping wherever becoming stuporous.

External control skill training supplies family members with information regarding maladaptive roles, eg. mascot, enabler, lost child, etc. The family then identifies in occupational therapy, through group processing and projective techniques, the maladaptive roles that each has assumed. For instance, a child asked to draw the family engaging in an activity, may inadvertently sketch the self away from the others, using light lines that denote the invisible characteristics of the "lost child." In discussing the drawing with the occupational therapist and the other family members, the child is helped to express feelings of isolation, fear and loneliness. The rest of the family becomes acutely aware of the need to help this child develop skills for interacting with others.

During the process of occupational therapy functional assessment, skills that each family member requires in order to relinquish maladaptive roles are determined. For example, a family member may state the desire to learn how to avoid arguments with the actively using substance abuser, a skill needed by the chief enabler and the scapegoat. The therapist and family delineate the components of the "argument-avoidance" skill (eg. firmly stating that the problem will be discussed at a time when the person is sober and then walking away from the intoxicated individual). The therapist models each skill component. Through role play, family members practice the skill components and receive feedback from each other and from other families. Barriers to skill implementation are identified and problem-solving is initiated to remove barriers when possible.

Changing Attitudes

At level one, the family expresses the years of anger generated by the substance abuser's behavior and disregard for the family's pain. Without this catharsis, the family has difficulty abandoning old, maladaptive roles and negative attitudes that served to perpetuate the addiction. Expressing unresolved anger in a passive-aggressive manner, or through blatant hostility directed toward the substance abuser, often creates family games, such as "Kick Me" or "Uproar."[21] The substance abuser uses family anger to further lower self-esteem and to provide corroborating evidence that "people are always picking on me." When the family agrees to "kick" the substance abuser, self-pity is an excellent reason to use drugs. The game of "Uproar" generates a shouting match over the least perceived infraction, thus justifying becoming intoxicated.

In order to avoid game playing in the future, the occupational therapist uses projective techniques that stimulate identification of anger and release of these emotions within the safe company of family members or other families who also experience similar feelings. Once feelings are identified and expressed, the family learns how these hostile, angry feelings contributed to the substance abuser's PDS. The key family attitudes promoting recovery are genuine concern, honesty and a nonjudgmental approach. The family determines alternative outlets for strong emotion until the substance abuser can adequately cope with the family's feelings. The family role plays and practices assertively expressing these feelings to the substance abuser in a manner that avoids blaming, is congruent with the situation, and is timed to correspond with periods of sobriety.[22]

Treatment Level Two

Separate groups or conjoint sessions with the substance abuser and the entire family may be indicated during treatment level two. The family goals for treatment level two emphasize coping and problem-solving. The family employs problem-solving techniques for all situations and not just those related to the substance abuser. Alternatives for coping are expanded that replace reliance on maladaptive roles. Strategies are developed that facilitate independent problem-solving and coping skills utilization.

The family and the substance abuser benefit from occupational therapy sessions focusing on assertiveness, stress management, cognitive-behavioral strategies, physical activity or biofeed-back. Planning for family weekend outings, designed as a means of spending time together and as a method of stress reduction, is an example of a joint occupational therapy session. The family is relearning how to play and have fun together now that family members can risk being genuine in each other's company. In terms of separate groups, the wife of the substance abuser, for instance, may want to develop assertive skills in order to respond to her husband's domineering tendencies that are no longer subdued by drugs.

By completion of treatment level two, the family and the substance abuser independently utilize newly learned coping skills. To ensure that transfer of coping skills from the treatment environment to the home results, the occupational therapist gives the substance abuser and the family increasing responsibility in selecting, planning and implementing their treatment goals. The family unit may decide, for instance, that parenting issues require emphasis in treatment. Parenting training assists the spouses in developing a united parental front. As a result, the parents help the children relinquish premature responsibilities assumed in response to the parents' past preoccupation with substance abuse.[23] Setting rules regarding curfews, limiting chores to more reasonable routines typical of the children's ages, and carefully responding to the children's resentment over lost control are examples of parental supervision skills learned in occupational therapy. Treatment for the children involves promoting roles more consistent with their ages, eg. playing, studying and dating.

Also contributing to the independence of the family, is the practicing of new family skills outside of occupational therapy groups according to specific "homework" assignments. For example, the daughter, who previously functioned as the family scapegoat, may contract with the occupational therapist to ask her father, who is recovering from substance abuse, to go to the movies with her as a means of improving the father-daughter relationship. In this way, family members gain experience with using problem-solving and coping skills in a variety of "real-life" circumstances. In addition, the substance abuser and the family are required to develop plans in occupational therapy that structure coping alternatives (eg. family meetings, family outings, leisure activities, shared family meals, etc.) into a daily schedule to be followed at home.

Treatment Level Three

The goals of treatment level three for the family involve emotional development and confrontation of maladaptive roles. Newly learned problem-solving skills are reinforced. Generalization of skills to a variety of situations is promoted. Family members relate to each other in a more mature fashion. Goals are set that focus the family on new directions for the future. In order to actually give up these maladaptive roles, the family members examine the way in which these roles met their own personal needs. This is accomplished in either separate or joint family sessions with the substance abuser depending on the therapeutic requirements of the situation.

In fact, the family learns that cessation of drug use could produce serious emotional upheaval.[24] Changes in life-style and family roles, even though an improvement over previous circumstances, are experienced as losses by the family.[25] Emotional development of each family member reorganizes the family system. When the family learns to focus on other important issues and problems, the substance abuser is removed from the center of attention; there is no longer someone upon whom to blame problems. Even though destructive, the old methods of responding to the intoxicated behavior were familiar and provided emotional security for the family.

Confrontation of continued reliance upon maladaptive roles by the family is the primary focus of the occupational therapy sessions. Occupational therapy sessions incorporate projective techniques and group processing methods that explore the family's need to maintain the individual's addiction. For example, during a collage activity designed to examine the wifes "payoff" in promoting her husband's addictive behavior, the wife discovers her persistent need "to be in charge."

Insight alone rarely results in behavioral changes.[26] Family members' self-discoveries are directed by the occupational therapist into problem-solving and implementation of coping strategies learned previously. To illustrate this, the wife from the previous example might solve problems regarding her control issues, such as assuming leadership in a group outside of the family and developing a plan with her husband to share family leadership. Thus, identified maladaptive role behaviors are changed into more satisfying styles of interacting, eg. no longer struggling with her husband for family power.

Then, the occupational therapist designs contexts in which maladaptive role behaviors were in the past typically elicited, eg. the wife's control issues surfaced when discussing family finances with her husband. The family experiences success in coping by instituting healthy role behaviors during situations that in the past produced maladaptive role behaviors (eg. the wife shares decision-making with her husband when paying the bills). Mosey refers to this process as "working through."[26] As a result, learning accumulated from the other two treatment levels is generalized to a variety of situations.

In addition to insight development and the working through process, goals for an "enabling-free" future are delineated in occupational therapy by each family member according to their respective interests and values. Occupational therapy facilitates family exploration of supporting values for healthy role development through values clarification, interests through interest surveys or the experiencing of potential interests, and skills through practice in carefully selected environments. For instance, the eldest child (the family hero) may decide to refocus his or her previous unrelenting pursuit of achievement by reorganizing time to include more leisure activities and fewer work-related activities. In doing so, the eldest child resolves the values conflict between engaging in leisure and viewing relaxation as "wasting time." Interesting leisure activities that accommodate abilities while simultaneously avoiding reinforcement of past over-achievement patterns, require identification.

◆ OUTCOMES ◆

Outcomes are the expected results of the interaction between PDS variables (substance abuser and family characteristics) and treatment variables, ie. PDS status, treatment levels, frames of reference and treatment methods (Table 8-6). General outcomes for the family are specified for each treatment level and include relinquished maladaptive role behavior at level one, improved coping at level two, and emotional development at level three.

Table 8-6
Treatment Outcomes

	Treatment Variables	+	PDS Variables	=	Outcomes
Level	Method	Frame of Reference	Addict/Family		Addict/Family
1	Directive	Behavioral	External control/ Relinquish enabling		Abstinence/Relinquished roles
2	Supportive	Cognitive	Internal control/ Develop coping		Improved coping
3	Confrontive	Object Relations	Insight/Stimulate growth		Emotional development

◆ CONCLUSIONS ◆

This chapter discussed the characteristics of the family that strongly influence treatment outcomes. Treatment variables that matched the characteristics of the family were described. Treatment methods were delineated for each treatment level. At level one, the family was taught how to live with the substance abuser. The family members were then taught how to live with themselves at treatment level two. Finally, at treatment level three, the family was taught how to live for the future. Outcomes of family therapy were delineated. It is hoped that this discussion prompts therapists to explore their role in the treatment of the family. This involvement of the family clearly augments the occupational therapy treatment program of the substance abuser.

References

1. Moyers PA: Occupational therapy intervention with the alcoholic's family. *Am J Occup Ther* 46(2): 105-111, 1992.
2. Moyers PA: Occupational therapy and treatment of the alcoholic's family. *Occup Ther Mental Health* 11(1): 45-64, 1991.
3. Moyers PA, Barrett CE: Treating the alcoholic's family. *Mental Health Special Interest Section Newsletter* 13(3): 2-4, 1990.
4. Hinojosa J: How mothers of preschool children with cerebral palsy perceive occupational and physical therapists and their influence on family life. *Occup Ther J Res* 10(3): 144-161, 1990.
5. Hinojosa J, Anderson J, Ranum GW: Relationships between therapists and parents of preschool children with cerebral palsy: A survey. *Occup Ther J Res* 8(5): 285-297, 1988.
6. Olson L, Heaney C, Soppas-Hoffman B: Parent-child activity group treatment in preventive psychiatry. *Occup Ther Health Care* 6(1): 29-43, 1989.
7. Petersen P, Wikoff RL: Home environment and adjustment in families with handicapped children: A canonical correlation study. *Occup Ther J Res* 7(2): 67-81, 1987.
8. Hasselkus BR: The meaning of daily activity in family caregiving for the elderly. *Am J Occup Ther* 43(10): 649-656, 1989.
9. Hasselkus BR: Ethical dilemmas in family caregiving for the elderly: Implications for occupational therapy. *Am J Occup Ther* 45(3): 206-212, 1991.
10. Gooderham M: The therapy of relationships. *Addictions* 19(4): 58-62, 1972.
11. Sedgwick R: *Family Mental Health Theory and Practice*. St. Louis, MO: C. V. Mosby Co, 1981.
12. Wegscheider D, Wegscheider S: *Family Illness: Chemical Dependency*. Minneapolis, MN: Johnson Institute, 1975.
13. Wegscheider S: From the family trap to family freedom. *Alcoholism* 1(3): 36-39, 1981.
14. Jacob T, Leonard, KE: Alcoholic-spouse interaction as a function of alcoholism subtype and alcohol consumption interaction. *J Abnorm Psychol* 97(2): 231-237, 1988.
15. Black C, Bucky SF, Wilder-Padilla S: The interpersonal and emotional consequences of being an adult child of an alcoholic. *Int J Addict* 21(2): 213-231, 1986.
16. Whitfield CL: Co-alcoholism: Recognizing a treatable illness. *Fam Comm Health* August: 16-27, 1984.
17. Cermak TL, Hunt T, Keene B, Thomas W: Codependency: More than a catchword. *Patient Care* August 15: 131-150, 1989.
18. Steinglass P: An experimental treatment program for alcoholic couples. *J Stud Alcohol* 40(3): 159-181, 1979.
19. Bluhm J: *When You Face the Chemically Dependent Patient: A Practical Guide for Nurses*. St. Louis, MO: Ishiyaku EuroAmerica, Inc., 1987.
20. Finley B: The family and substance abuse. In Bennett G, Vourakis C, & Woolf D (Eds.): *Substance Abuse: Pharmacologic, Developmental, and Clinical Perspectives*. New York: John Wiley & Sons, 1983.
21. Steiner C: *Games Alcoholics Play*. New York: Grove Press, 1971.
22. Satir V, Stachowiak J, Taschman HA: *Helping Families to Change*. Northvale, NJ: Jason Aronson, Inc., 1983.
23. Fox R: *The Effect of Alcoholism on Children*. New York: National Council on Alcoholism, 1972.
24. McCabe TR: *Victims No More*. Center City, MN: Hazelden, 1978.
25. Swift HA, Williams T: *Recovery For the Whole Family*. Center City, MN: Hazelden, 1975.
26. Mosey AC: *Psychosocial Components of Occupational Therapy*. New York: Raven Press, 1986.

Sandra
A Case Example

INTRODUCTION

This chapter illustrates the occupational therapy
treatment principles for substance abusers. A case study
is presented that begins with referral to an inpatient
occupational therapy program and follows the progression of the substance abuser through the three treatment
level. A structured occupational therapy aftercare program is included as part of the case.

Screening is demonstrated along with initial frame
of reference determination. Treatment planning, including the selection of appropriate treatment methods, is
conducted with the substance abuser at the beginning of
each treatment level. Monitoring the substance abuser's
recovery process is illustrated so that the importance of
evaluating ongoing changes in the PDS status is
understood. Frame of reference changes occur with
progression to successive treatment levels. Sample
patient documentation is presented. Involvement of the
family in the occupational therapy treatment program is
demonstrated as well.

◆ SCREENING ◆

REFERRAL AND CHART REVIEW

The occupational therapist received a referral for a female alcoholic, Sandra Jones, hospitalized for the first time in an inpatient substance abuse rehabilitation facility. The referral from the facility's medical director stated "evaluate level of functional independence and begin treatment as indicated." After receipt of referral, the occupational therapist completed a chart review with the results contained in Figure 9-1.

Name ___Sandra Jones___ **Age** ___34___ **Date** ___8/31/93___

Occupational Therapy Referral Date ___8/31/93___
Referring Physician ___Dr. Adams___ **Admission Date** ___8/30/93___
Diagnosis ___Alcohol dependence___

Medications ___Librium to control withdrawal and multivitamins.___

Reason for Admission ___Husband threatened divorce if patient did not stop drinking.___

Presenting Problems ___Stopped drinking two days prior to admission. Patient reports anxiety, insomnia, headaches, depressed mood, suicidal thoughts and motor restlessness.___

Drinking History ___Drinking vodka approximately 5xs/wk for the last year, drinks until passes out, drinks alone after husband goes to work, sneaking and hiding alcohol, occasional blackouts (reported by husband).___

Previous Psychiatric History ___None___

Mental Status ___Pt. was well dressed upon admission, was restless, exhibited underlying hostility, & speech was guarded as pt. gave brief answers to questions. Mood was sad, affect was angry but appropriate to situation. No hallucinations, stream of thought was adequate, no thought disturbances, oriented Xs 3, completed serial 7s, memory and abstract reasoning intact, good judgment and demonstrated insight, but denied being alcoholic.___

Family History ___Married 10 years. Not able to have children. Husband drinks socially. Pt. reported father as being an alcoholic.___

Education ___One semester of college___ **Work** ___Housewife___

Precautions/Complications ___Suicidal, smokes cigarettes, AK amputation of right leg resulting from bone cancer in 1986. Uses a crutch for mobility.___

PDS Variables ___Alcohol dependence, loss of control over drinking; denies alcohol as a problem; depressed mood; support system limited to husband (no friends); stress from possible divorce, past history of cancer and being infertile; limited satisfying roles; unresolved issues related to father's drinking.___

PDS Status ___Treatment level 1___

Figure 9-1. Occupational therapy chart review.

Based on the chart information, the occupational therapist listed pertinent PDS variables which included alcohol dependence; loss of control over drinking; denial of alcohol as a problem; depressed mood; support system limited to husband; stressors of possible divorce, past history of cancer, and infertility; and limited satisfying roles. Comparisons of these variables to Table 4-3, Chart Data and Corresponding PDS Variables, led to the conclusion that the patient would benefit from treatment level one strategies. An interview and performance assessment were conducted to corroborate the PDS status determination.

INTERVIEW

The occupational therapist utilized the Occupational Case Analysis Interview and Rating Scale (OCAIRS) to collect data indicating present functioning and current PDS status.[1] Figure 9-2 contains the results. Level one PDS status was upheld. Denial of alcohol and rationalizing drinking as resulting from depression indicated need for treatment level one. Gaps in Sandra's daily schedule illustrated the strong influence of daily drinking upon current lifestyle.

Additional PDS variables were ascertained from the interview. The interview highlighted Sandra's passivity and dependence upon her husband. Sandra had not solved problems regarding access to transportation and had become increasingly isolated from others. As a result, Sandra depended upon her husband for social interaction and to transport her as needed. Of further concern was the role of Sandra's husband in promoting dependency and enabling the alcoholism. This problem required further exploration. While Sandra was unable to go shopping due to lack of transportation, she had access to a supply of liquor. Based on the interview, it was determined that Sandra was using alcohol to cope with boredom and social isolation.

The interview ascertained specific strengths that were useful in treatment. Cognitive functioning was intact, at least in terms of verbal interaction and past history of cognitive performance, ie, receiving As in two college courses. Also, Sandra demonstrated insight by expressing dissatisfaction with current occupational performance. She verbalized awareness of life stressors, ie. cancer, infertility and growing up with a drinking parent. Sandra valued her relationship with her husband, which motivated her interest in making changes. Also noteworthy was Sandra's desire to obtain further education and to develop career opportunities.

PERFORMANCE MEASURE

Due to limited time for the evaluation and because Sandra expressed a desire to attend the occupational therapy craft group, it was decided to observe Sandra's task performance using The Comprehensive Occupational Therapy Evaluation Scale (COTE Scale).[2] Figure 9-3 contains the information and substantiates the impressions formulated from the chart review and the interview. New insights were also gained.

During the hour long craft group, Sandra worked on a wooden mug holder. Personal appearance was neat and clean and Sandra came to the group on time without any reminders. Sandra selected a task without hesitation and began work, requiring no encouragement to initiate the activity. Fine motor coordination was somewhat affected by a slight tremulousness of the hands. Sandra was irritated by this tremor and became frustrated when trying to stencil the mug rack. There was no evidence of bizarre behavior and pacing on task was within normal limits. Affect was appropriate to the situation, but mood was generally sad. Sandra demonstrated responsibility for errors made on the task (ie. not blaming others for mistakes) and for maintaining the neatness of the occupational therapy clinic.

Cognitive skills were intact as demonstrated by Sandra's ability to concentrate on the

Patient	Sandra
OT Rater	Penny Moyers
Date	9/28/93

(Adaptive 5 4 3 2 1 Maladaptive)		
Personal Causation	4	Runs household, frustrated with career plans, completed one semester of college. Depressed.
Values and Goals	4	Values marriage; wants to continue college majoring in accounting and gain control of depression.
Interests	3	Housework, soap operas, dancing. Rarely goes dancing; husband works 2nd shift and AK amputation.
Roles	4	Housewife (cooking, cleaning, laundry, pays bills). Husband helps her shop as she doesn't drive.
Habits	2	Organized around soap opera schedule. Cooks dinner around 3:00 pm before husband goes to work.
Skills	4	Housekeeping skills adequate. Fighting with husband. No friends. Husband makes decisions.
Output	2	Bored; lonely; not able to meet people.
Physical	2	Unable to drive due to R AK amputation. No bus transportation available. Lives in isolated area.
Social Environment	3	Husband wants her to stop drinking. Denies drinking. States feels depressed.
Feedback	2	Feels like killing herself; crying constantly. Husband wants divorce if she doesn't stop drinking.
Dynamic	3	Output minimal; few interests; not proud of ability. Abstinence not a current goal.
Historical	2	Cancer, infertility, alcoholic father. Felt life better before having cancer and when newly married.
Contextual	2	Environment supports college. Needs friends and to resolve transportation problems.
Trajectory	2	In a reoccurring maladaptive cycle.

Figure 9-2. OCAIRS Occupational Case Analysis Interview and Rating Scale results: Summary form. *From Kaplan K, Kielhofner G: Occupational Case Analysis Interview and Rating Scale. Thorofare, NJ: Slack, Inc., 1989, p. 15. Reprinted with permission.*

task for 20 minute periods without a break or without redirection from the therapist. Sandra followed verbal and written directions, recognized and solved minor problems, and learned a moderately complex activity quickly. Initial interest was shown in the activity and in finishing the task according to personal standards. However, Sandra was overly critical of her performance and seemed to set high standards for herself. Sandra had difficulty dealing with frustration as noted by an increase in self-depreciating remarks. These negative self-statements occurred after committing errors due to coordination difficulties. Interest in

Date	$^{9}/_{28}$														
I. General Behavior	1	2	3	4	5	6	7	8	9	10	11	12	13	14	15
A. Appearance	0														
B. Non-productive behavior	4														
C. Activity level (a or b)	0														
D. Expression	4														
E. Responsibility	0														
F. Punctuality	0														
G. Reality orientation	0														
II. Interpersonal Behavior	1	2	3	4	5	6	7	8	9	10	11	12	13	14	15
A. Engagement	0														
B. Cooperation	2														
C. Self-assertion (a or b)	2														
D. Sociability	4														
E. Attention-getting behavior	0														
F. Negative response from others	4														
G. Reaction to authority figure	0														
III. Task Behavior	1	2	3	4	5	6	7	8	9	10	11	12	13	14	15
A. Engagement	0														
B. Concentration	0														
C. Coordination	1														
D. Follow directions	0														
E. Activity neatness or attention to detail	0														
F. Problem-solving	1														
G. Complexity and organization of task	0														
H. Initial learning	0														
I. Interest in activity	0														
J. Interest in accomplishment	0														
K. Decision-making	0														
L. Frustration tolerance	4														

Scale: 0 - Normal,   1 - Minimal,   2 - Mild,   3 - Moderate,   4 - Severe

DATES		IDENTIFIED PROBLEM AREAS	(Therapist's Signature)
Identified	**Resolved**		
9/28/93		Nonproductive behavior – Preoccupied with own thoughts	
9/28/93		Expression – Uncontrolled expression when frustrated	
9/28/93		Cooperation – Became oppositional when frustrated, aggressive when angry	
9/28/93		Sociability – Does not join others in activities	
9/28/93		Negative response – Evokes numerous negative responses	
9/28/93		Coordination – Tremulous frustration tolerance; high self-expectations	

Figure 9-3. COTE results. *From Brayman S, et al.: Comprehensive occupational therapy evaluation scale. Am J Occup Ther 30(2): 94-100. Reprinted with permission.*

completing the task changed once errors were made. At this point, Sandra cleaned up the area and requested to return to her room.

The main difficulties according to the COTE Scale were related to interpersonal behaviors. Sandra was independent in task performance, but failed to ask for help when encountering difficulties. She was cooperative with the therapist until wanting to leave the group early. She also ignored others in the room, even when asked by another patient to provide assistance. Sandra responded to this request by stating, "you'll have to figure it out for yourself....I can't help you." Generally, Sandra did not talk to others and gave brief responses when questions were directed to her. She isolated herself from the rest of the group by working at a table that was away from most of the group members.

DATA SYNTHESIS

Based on the chart review, interview and performance measure, it was determined that Sandra required treatment level one intervention. Figure 9-4 presents a list of tentative problems and strengths synthesized from the data. Notice the differentiation between functional problems and component dysfunctions. These strengths and problems were used to formulate the tentative occupational therapy functional diagnosis.

The major role problems were marital discord and few occupational roles. Performance dysfunction was indicated by Sandra's impoverished daily routine and inability to drive. Component dysfunction, contributing to the functional impairments, included loss of control over drinking, denial of alcoholism, experiencing multiple stressors, coping with alcohol, restricted social support, interpersonal skills deficits and depressed mood. The above-the-knee amputation of the right lower extremity and living in an isolated geographic area severely limited her transportation options.

Numerous strengths were identified as role, performance and component functioning. In terms of role and performance functioning, Sandra described intact housekeeping skills and corresponding adequate role performance in this area. She also demonstrated a neat appearance, indicating intact ADL performance skills. The most important component functioning involved intact cognitive skills and values related to marriage, career and education. The chart review, OCAIRS and the COTE scale provided cues contributing to the occupational therapy diagnosis.[1,2] The role, performance and component dysfunctions were related to the pathology of alcohol dependence.

FRAME OF REFERENCE SELECTION

From the occupational therapy functional diagnosis, an occupational therapy frame of reference was chosen that was appropriate for treatment level one intervention. Because cognitive skills were intact, management of cognitive disabilities was not considered appropriate. It was desirable to choose a frame of reference that would be useful for treatment level two. The expectation was for this patient to progress rapidly to treatment level two due to cognitive abilities, initial level of insight and desire to save her marriage.

The model of human occupation was selected due to the need for PDS mobilization. It was important for Sandra to analyze the impact of drinking upon her role and performance functioning. The model of human occupation easily makes the transition to treatment level two when Sandra is ready. The model of human occupation will be helpful in resolving treatment level two issues of dependency and passivity which ultimately influence successful problem-solving and coping in occupational roles.

Strengths

Role/Performance Functioning:
1. Intact housekeeping skills
2. Intact grooming/hygiene skills

Component Functioning:
1. Intact cognitive skills
2. Values related to marriage, career, and education

Problems

Role/Performance Dysfunction:
1. Deterioration of marital relationship (max assist to interact with husband without arguments)
2. Impoverishment of daily routine (max assist to reorganize daily routine)
3. Limited number of roles (max assist to increase number of satisfying roles)
4. Totally dependent in transportation in the community.

Component Dysfunction (underlying factors); (max assist required to resolve):
1. Denial of alcoholism
2. Lack of support system
3. Few interests
4. Interpersonal skills deficit
5. Multiple stressors
6. No independent transportation
7. Low frustration tolerance
8. Drinking to cope
9. Perfectionistic
10. Dependent on husband
11. Passivity (problem-solving)
12. Depressed mood
13. Unresolved issues regarding father's drinking

Cues OCAIRS indicated few roles, vague daily routine, depression, and denial of alcoholism. COTE Scale showed task performance impaired by perfectionism, low frustration tolerance, and impaired interpersonal skills.

Pathology   Alcohol dependence

Functional Prognosis Based on intact cognitive skills, articulated values and goals, insight regarding stressors, and past history of successful functional performance, the prognosis is excellent for Sandra to achieve the occupational therapy treatment level 1 goals.

Figure 9-4. Tentative problem list.

◆ TREATMENT LEVEL ONE ◆

OCCUPATIONAL THERAPY ASSESSMENT

After selecting the frame of reference, the occupational therapist could either finalize the treatment level one functional status or could proceed with in depth evaluation if not enough pertinent data were obtained. The occupational therapist determined that enough data were gathered and therefore specified the diagnosis in order to guide treatment level one treatment planning. Figure 9-5 outlines the treatment level one diagnosis.

Role Dysfunction	Few satisfying roles. Moderate assist needed to acknowledge influence of drinking on role performance.
Performance Dysfunction	Impoverished daily routine. Moderate assist in recognizing behaviors associated with onset of drinking.
Component Dysfunction	Denial of alcoholism, restricted support system, low frustration tolerance, perfectionism, and depressed mood.
Cues	OCAIRS indicated few roles, vague daily routine, depression, and denial of alcoholism. COTE Scale showed task performance impaired by perfectionism, low frustration tolerance, and impaired interpersonal skills.
Pathology	Alcohol dependence.

Figure 9-5. Treatment level one diagnosis.

Not enough time had elapsed to note functional changes attributable to detoxification. The functional prognosis was based on intact cognitive skills, articulated values and goals, insight regarding stressors and past history of successful functional performance. The prognosis was excellent for Sandra to achieve the occupational therapy treatment level one goals.

TREATMENT PLANNING

The occupational therapist met with Sandra to plan the course of treatment (Figure 9-6). The treatment plan focused on treatment level one issues and was expected to be completed in two weeks. After two weeks, the occupational therapist met with Sandra to determine readiness for treatment level two and to develop goals and methods appropriate for that treatment level.

Because of Sandra's intact cognitive abilities and motivation for treatment, the occupational therapist included Sandra in the treatment planning process. The occupational therapist began the planning session by explaining to Sandra the results of the evaluation and the corresponding functional diagnosis. Sandra gave feedback regarding the relevancy of the occupational therapy diagnosis. Based on this give-and-take interaction, the diagnosis was accepted. The occupational therapist was careful to equally emphasize the strengths and the weaknesses, monitoring any strong negative responses. The occupational therapist and Sandra agreed on the goals and the treatment methods.

A substance abuser who strongly denies drug use may react negatively to the treatment planning session, consequently destroying rapport. The occupational therapist uses professional judgment to determine the substance abuser's ego strength for tolerating treatment planning. This assessment of ego strength incorporates knowledge of PDS principles, especially in regards to confrontation. Joint treatment planning may be postponed until denial is not as strong. In some cases, treatment planning is modified so that only level of participation in occupational therapy is determined or only one problem is discussed at a time.

TREATMENT IMPLEMENTATION

Treatment goals were selected that corresponded with PDS issues. The first two weeks were spent on challenging denial of alcoholism. In this regard, the occupational therapist encouraged Sandra to connect current social isolation and role dissatisfaction with the influence of drinking.

Name _____Sandra Jones_____**Date**_____9/1/93_____ **PDS Status** _Level 1_

Functional Problems _Deterioration of marital relationship, impoverishment of daily routine and_ limited number of roles.

Underlying Factors
1. Denial of alcoholism
2. Lack of support system
3. Low frustration tolerance
4. Perfectionistic
5. Depressed mood (suicidal)

Strengths
1. Cognitive skills
2. Career goals (accountant)
3. Educational goal (obtain college degree)
4. Values marriage

Goals

LTG 1: Sandra will with min assist engage in a selected interest that replaces time originally spent in drinking (2 weeks).

    STG 1a: Week one, Sandra will determine with mod assist the effect of drinking on her routine.

    STG 1b: Week one, Sandra will identify with min assist gaps in schedule available to activities of interest.

    STG 1c: Week one, Sandra will select with mod assist satisfying interests that replace time spent in drinking.

    STG 1d: Week two, Sandra will express with min assist relationship between sobriety and future successes in engagement in satisfying interests.

LTG 2: Sandra will no longer exhibit with min assist behaviors previously associated with onset of drinking episodes during engagement in selected interests (2 weeks).

    STG 2a: Week one, Sandra will identify with mod assist behaviors that precede drinking.

    STG 2b: Week two, Sandra will implement with min assist biofeedback to control frustration.

Method _3 individual sessions per/wk. for 2 weeks for biofeedback training and for goal progress_ assessment. Attend daily for two weeks the Lifestyles Group and 2Xs/wk for 2 weeks the Interest Exploration Group.

Figure 9-6. Occupational therapy treatment plan.

Principles of selective denial required the avoidance of exploring other factors contributing to social isolation and role dissatisfaction, eg. passivity, dependence, unresolved issues regarding a drinking parent, etc. Denial of the effects of drinking was also challenged when Sandra examined the negative behaviors closely associated with drinking episodes. Specifically, those behaviors observed in occupational therapy, such as perfectionism, low frustration tolerance and depressed mood, were targeted for change.

Sober rationalization was also reflected in the treatment plan. Short-term goal "1d" expected Sandra to delineate the impact of sobriety upon future successes in terms of engaging in self-selected interests. In this way, Sandra created positive associations with sobriety that motivated her to achieve abstinence. The Interest Exploration Group (craft group) allowed Sandra to experience successes related to activity performance and sober control of behavior.

Other PDS mobilization techniques are not as clearly evident in the treatment plan, but were implied either through the goals or through the treatment methods. For instance, assimilative projection was fostered in the Lifestyles Group. Group members discerned the impact of drinking upon their lifestyles. In this way, Sandra learned that she was not the only one that had problems as the result of drinking. Assimilative projection was necessary to combat Sandra's social isolation and to lay the foundation for interpersonal skills development.

Another important PDS factor was the subtle switch from passive modes of problem-solving to more active involvement. After identifying some behaviors that triggered the desire to drink, Sandra was given a method of controlling these feelings through biofeedback. Sandra identified these triggering behaviors in both the Lifestyle Group and in the Interest Exploration Group. In the Lifestyle Group, Sandra looked at past trigger behaviors by describing events and feelings that occurred prior to drinking episodes. In the Interest Exploration group, Sandra assessed current trigger behaviors. During craft group, (Interest Exploration) sessions, the occupational therapist helped Sandra modify frustration tolerance and perfectionism at the time that these behaviors occurred. A transition from reliance on external control to developing internal control was occurring. Sandra, as a result, was prepared for the aggressive development of coping skills that is characteristic of treatment level two.

Biofeedback also reduced Sandra's tendency to attribute detoxification symptom improvement (headaches, tremors, anxiety, depression, insomnia, etc.) as being the result of Librium. The therapist prompted Sandra to give biofeedback credit for control of the symptoms as well. The individual biofeedback treatment sessions and the weekly progress sessions also mobilized the PDS through sober selective attention. The occupational therapist redirected obsession with alcohol to sobriety. This was accomplished by reinforcing Sandra's efforts to produce abstinence behaviors with one-to-one attention from the therapist. The structured treatment schedule accommodated desire for predictability. Reliance on dichotomous behavioral responses was offset by involvement in a structured daily routine.

REEVALUATION AND DOCUMENTATION

In Sandra's case, progress was assessed in three ways. The COTE Scale documented behavioral changes in the Interest Exploration group.[2] The COTE Scale compared one rating period to the next. Figure 9-7 contains the COTE Scale with ratings completed after the first and second weeks of therapy. Biofeedback's influence on anxiety was determined by pre- and post-testing on the Spielberger's State-Trait Anxiety Scale.[3]

The other method of progress assessment involved meeting with Sandra in order to formulate conclusions regarding goal attainment and readiness for treatment level advancement. The initial treatment plan required Sandra and the occupational therapist to meet after the first week of treatment and then again after the second week of treatment. The occupational therapist wrote progress notes weekly to communicate results of the reevaluation measures to the treatment team. Figure 9-8 contains the second progress note completed after two weeks of therapy.

◆ TREATMENT LEVEL TWO ◆

OCCUPATIONAL THERAPY ASSESSMENT

With the decision to progress to treatment level two, the occupational therapist selected specific measures to examine coping skill baseline status. The Gambrill-Richey Assertion Inventory indicated lack of assertive skills.[4] The COPE Inventory of Coping Skills suggested a general lack of coping skills other than using alcohol to combat stress.[5] Sandra described biofeedback techniques

Date	9/29	10/5	10/12												
I. General Behavior	1	2	3	4	5	6	7	8	9	10	11	12	13	14	15
A. Appearance	0	0	0												
B. Non-productive behavior	4	3	1												
C. Activity level (a or b)	0	0	0												
D. Expression	4	2	0												
E. Responsibility	0	0	0												
F. Punctuality	0	0	0												
G. Reality orientation	0	0	0												
II. Interpersonal Behavior	1	2	3	4	5	6	7	8	9	10	11	12	13	14	15
A. Engagement	0	0	0												
B. Cooperation	2	2	1												
C. Self-assertion (a or b)	2	1	0												
D. Sociability	4	3	2												
E. Attention-getting behavior	0	0	0												
F. Negative response from others	4	3	2												
G. Reaction to authority figure	0	0	0												
III. Task Behavior	1	2	3	4	5	6	7	8	9	10	11	12	13	14	15
A. Engagement															
B. Concentration	0	0	0												
C. Coordination	0	0	0												
D. Follow directions	1	0	0												
E. Activity neatness or attention to detail	0	0	0												
F. Problem-solving	0	0	0												
G. Complexity and organization of task	1	0	0												
H. Initial learning	0	0	0												
I. Interest in activity	0	0	0												
J. Interest in accomplishment	0	0	0												
K. Decision-making	0	0	0												
L. Frustration tolerance	4	3	2												

Scale: 0 = Normal,   1 = Minimal,   2 = Mild,   3 = Moderate,   4 = Severe

DATES		IDENTIFIED PROBLEM AREAS	(Therapist's Signature)
Identified	**Resolved**		
9/28/93		Nonproductive behavior – Preoccupied with own thoughts	
9/28/93	10/12/93	Expression – Uncontrolled expression when frustrated	
9/28/93	Assertion 10/12/93	Cooperation – Oppositional when frustrated; aggressive when angry	
9/28/93		Sociability – Does not join others in activities	
9/28/93		Negative response – Evokes numerous negative responses	
9/28/93	Coordination 10/5	Coordination – Tremulous frustration tolerance; high self-expectation	

Figure 9-7. COTE first and second week results. *From Brayman S, et al.: Comprehensive occupational therapy evaluation scale. Am J Occup Ther 30(2): 94-100. Reprinted with permission.*

Name   Sandra Jones   **Date**   9/15/93

S: "I realize that I had a drinking problem for a long time. I just didn't want to admit it. My husband knew all along, but didn't know how to help me. I know I hurt him, but I feel good about being able to change things."

O: Sandra completed two weeks of occupational therapy including 2 individual sessions, 4 biofeedback training sessions, 4 Interest Exploration Group sessions, and 10 lifestyle Group sessions. Since last progress notation on 9/9/93, COTE Scale and anxiety reevaluations were conducted to determine progress on goals. See the evaluation section of the chart for further details.

Results of the reevaluations indicate that Sandra has significantly reduced anxiety level and is able to implement biofeedback strategies independently as needed without reminders from therapist. In the Lifestyle Group, Sandra examined her normal routine, noting time previously spent in drinking and the need to reorganize her schedule. Sandra verbalized influence of drinking on social role performance, marital relationship, and activity output. During the Interest Exploration Group, Sandra is engaging in self-identified interests independently. Incidence of perfectionism and low frustration tolerance affecting task performance has decreased. Sandra still requires moderate assistance from therapist to control these behaviors. Sandra also does not recognize behaviors other than perfectionism and low frustration tolerance as contributing to urges to drink. Interactions with others have shown improvement (initiates conversation and no longer isolates self from others) and Sandra is now ready to begin work on interpersonal skill development.

A: The status on the goals are as follows:

LTG 1: Sandra will with min assist engage in selected interest that replaces time originally   D/C 9/15/93
spent in drinking (2 weeks).

    STG 1a: Week one, Sandra will determine with mod assist the effect of drinking on   D/C 9/15/93
    her routine.

    STG 1b: Week one, Sandra will identify with min assist gaps in schedule available   D/C 9/15/93
    to activities of interest.

    STG 1c: Week one, Sandra will select with mod assist satisfying interests that   D/C 9/15/93
    replace time spent in drinking.

    STG 1d: Week two, Sandra will express with min assist relationship between   D/C 9/15/93
    sobriety and future successes in engagement in satisfying interests.

LTG 2: Sandra will no longer exhibit with min assist behaviors previously associated with   cont 9/29/93
onset of drinking episodes during engagement in selected interests (2 weeks).

    STG 2a: Week one, Sandra will identify with mod assist behaviors that precede   cont 9/29/93
    drinking.

    STG 2b: Week two, Sandra will implement with min assist biofeedback to control   D/C 9/15/93
    frustration.

P: In addition to continuing with LTG 2 and STG 2a, the following goals as agreed upon with Sandra will be implemented:

    STG 2c: By discharge, Sandra will identify independently coping strategies for major stressors.

    STG 2d: By discharge, Sandra will incorporate with standby assist three new coping strategies into daily routine.

    STG 2e: By discharge, Sandra will demonstrate 75% of the time with standby assist assertive behavior during interactions with others.

Method: Interpersonal Skills Group 3Xs/wk, Stress Management Group 2Xs/wk for 2 weeks, and referral to Driving Rehabilitation Program at General Hospital. Interest Exploration Group and Lifestyle Group will be discontinued.

Figure 9-8. Occupational therapy progress (SOAP) note. S=Subjective; O=Objective; A= Assessment; P=Plan.

as a possible coping strategy but lacked confidence in her ability to use this strategy at home when significantly stressed. Rotter's I-E Locus of Control Scale showed a slight external orientation.[6]

The occupational therapy functional status was reformulated to reflect the specific issues of treatment level two. Figure 9-9 outlines the rewritten occupational therapy diagnosis.

The functional status of Sandra was further described by outlining the functional changes occurring upon completion of treatment level one. As indicated previously, the major change was in denial. Sandra recognized influence of alcohol upon past and future role and performance functioning. Sandra reported successes in using biofeedback to control anxiety and in reducing frustration levels. Because of excellent progress made in confronting denial and in articulating desire to cope differently, it was expected that Sandra would achieve the goals for treatment level two.

Role Dysfunction	Few satisfying roles and impaired marital relationship.
Performance Dysfunction	Impoverished daily routine. Needs moderate assist to identify and incorporate interests and alternative coping strategies in the daily routine.
Component Dysfunction	Coping skills limited to Biofeedback. Lacks assertive skills. Dependent upon husband to make decisions and to provide transportation. Needs moderate assist to communicate needs to husband.
Cues	Gambrill-Richey Assertion Inventory indicates lack of assertive skills. COPE Inventory shows coping limited to alcohol and biofeedback. Lack of efficacy regarding use of biofeedback.
Pathology	Alcohol dependence.

Figure 9-9. Occupational therapy level two diagnosis.

FRAME OF REFERENCE

Initially, the model of human occupation was selected to guide level one treatment. This frame of reference remained relevant at treatment level two. The model of human occupation was selected due to its emphasis upon coping and developing an internal sense of control during occupational role performance. Cognitive-behavioral techniques were used to promote internal control and to develop communication skills necessary for role functioning. Cognitive-behavioral techniques focus on the correction of faulty conceptions and self-signals that affect functional performance.[7]

Emotions are viewed by cognitive theory as a consequence of negative thinking triggered by an unsuccessful experience.[7] The substance abuser analyzes negative emotions by determining the event that produced the emotion and highlighting the negative self-talk that ultimately occurs. Strategies are taught to change the negative thoughts to more positive thoughts. This is followed by constructive action, taken during role activities, that reinforces the changed thought structure and the resulting positive emotions.

TREATMENT PLANNING

As indicated by the progress note in Figure 9-8, Sandra was ready for treatment level two. The main improvement was in denial. Sandra admitted that drinking was a significant problem in her life. Furthermore, Sandra still needed to work on interpersonal skills. Additionally, Sandra needed to develop coping abilities and confidence in employing them independently during times of stress. Similar to the first treatment planning session, the occupational therapist met with Sandra to delineate treatment goals and methods consistent with the revised diagnosis. The main difference in this treatment planning session and the first session was that Sandra took more control in terms of delineating problems and treatment methods.

TREATMENT IMPLEMENTATION

The revised treatment plan indicates the switch in emphasis from PDS mobilization to developing alternative strategies to cope with stress. These alternative strategies weaken over-reliance on the PDS. Sandra was referred to the Interpersonal Skills group where assertive behaviors were taught and practiced. The Stress Management Group identified major stressors and developed methods to reduce stress without using alcohol. The Stress Management Group began where the biofeedback training ended. Note also the referral to a driving rehabilitation program. Transporting the self independently would decrease Sandra's social isolation and dependency on her husband.

FAMILY INVOLVEMENT

Treatment level two was the appropriate time to include participation by Sandra's husband, Mike, in occupational therapy. There were several methods for accomplishing this objective. Sandra identified in group specific relationship tasks to work on with her husband during visiting hours or during weekend passes home. For example, Sandra expressed concern in the assertiveness training group about not spending enough time in enjoyable leisure activities with her husband. While she was drinking, Mike occupied himself in interests that helped him avoid facing Sandra's drinking problem. Without intervention, Mike would probably continue this solitary activity, even though Sandra might no longer be drinking.

Sandra expressed in group her fear of asking Mike to do something special with her during her next weekend pass. The Interpersonal Skills Group encouraged Sandra, after practicing through role playing, to assertively ask Mike to change his plans to include activities they could share together. After following through on the assignment, Sandra reported back to the group the successes and the difficulties in accomplishing her assertiveness objective. Eventually, Sandra assertively made decisions regarding how her time was to be spent on weekend passes. Her planning allotted time for her and Mike to engage in joint activities together. Sandra also developed interests that she could independently experience without Mike. The last several sessions of the Interpersonal Skills Group incorporated direct participation by select family members. The family experimented with assertive communication noting the influence upon family system dynamics.

REEVALUATION

Prior to discharge from the inpatient occupational therapy program, Sandra and the occupational therapist met to ascertain progress on the goals that were added to the treatment plan. The inpatient occupational therapist reevaluated Sandra's assertiveness skills, general coping ability and internal versus external orientation. Pre- and post-tests were compared using the Gambrill-Richey Assertion Inventory, the COPE Inventory of Coping Skills, and the Rotter's I-E Locus of Control Scale.[4-6]

On all measures, Sandra's scores indicated improvement. The most significant change was on the I-E Locus of Control Scale which indicated a much stronger internal orientation.[6] Progress was also reported from the rehabilitation driver's program. Sandra mastered the compensatory techniques in manipulating the gas and brake pedals with the left lower extremity. She was preparing to complete her driver's test in order to obtain her license. These objective measures indicated readiness for treatment level three. Sandra was demonstrating the ego strength necessary to resolve some of the issues of the addiction.

◆ TREATMENT LEVEL THREE ◆

OCCUPATIONAL THERAPY ASSESSMENT

The occupational therapist, with Sandra's permission, consulted the aftercare occupational therapist in selecting treatment level three evaluation tools. This, of course, assumed that the occupational therapist conducting the aftercare program was one who communicated with the inpatient therapist and was willing to continue the occupational therapy program begun during inpatient hospitalization. In this case example, the aftercare occupational therapist worked for the same organization as the inpatient occupational therapist. Because the two occupational therapists worked for the same facility, treatment level three evaluation began prior to actual discharge from the inpatient substance abuse program. This strategy aided in the transition from one therapist to another and ensured continuity of Sandra's treatment.

The occupational therapist, in conjunction with the aftercare occupational therapist, selected The Problem Situation Inventory as a baseline measurement tool for evaluating Sandra's ability to independently cope with stressful relapse situations.[8] The Magazine Picture Collage facilitated discussion related to the issues of addiction and the pending discharge.[9] The Personal Orientation Inventory examined Sandra's ability to articulate values consistent with sobriety as well as her ability to utilize these values in decision making.[10] From these tools, the occupational therapy diagnosis was reformulated to reflect the problems of treatment level three. The diagnosis was jointly developed by the two occupational therapists (Figure 9-10).

The functional changes that occurred with treatment level two implementation indicated an excellent prognosis for treatment level three. Sandra demonstrated assertive skills and practiced a variety of coping strategies during stressful times experienced during the hospitalization. Little prompting from the therapist was required to facilitate healthy coping. Sandra was less passive in making decisions or in solving problems, thereby demonstrating a more internal locus of control.

FRAME OF REFERENCE

With the advent of treatment level three, a frame of reference addition was indicated. The model of human occupation aptly addressed the process of adding satisfying roles, ie. career and educational goals, to the daily routine. The emphasis in treatment upon meeting new people corresponded to the performance subsystem skill of communication/interaction. At issue,

Role Dysfunction	Few satisfying roles and impaired marital relationship. Needs minimal assist to express emotional issues with her husband. Needs moderate assist to explore career and educational opportunities.
Performance Dysfunction	Impoverished daily routine. Needs minimal assist to consistently implement interests and alternative coping strategies in the daily routine.
Component Dysfunction	Coping and assertive skills tenuous, requiring practice in real situations. Has not resolved issues related to father's drinking, infertility, and cancer.
Cues	Problem Situations Inventory indicates lack of self-confidence in ability to cope under significant stress. The Personal Orientation Inventory suggests that difficulty in articulating values may impede decision making. Projective testing highlights negative affect associated with unresolved issues that may interfere with adaptive coping.
Pathology	Alcohol dependence.

Figure 9-10. Occupational therapy level three diagnosis.

though, was exploring influences of past experiences upon current behavior. This did not fit with the principles of the model of human occupation.

Instead, the aftercare occupational therapist decided to also utilize the object relations frame of reference. There was a need to bring feelings regarding past stressors to the conscious level. It is not unusual for the occupational therapist to utilize more than one frame of reference at a time. Holm discussed the systems approach to frame of reference selection.[11] This approach involves choosing a frame(s) of reference that is appropriate for each specific problem. There was a need for frames of reference that were capable of focusing on two divergent issues. Thus, the object relations frame of reference helped Sandra become aware of unrecognized feelings related to unresolved stressful experiences. The model of human occupation was useful in developing new satisfying roles, communication/interaction skills, and instituting newly identified interests.

TREATMENT PLANNING

Once the diagnosis was reformulated, the two occupational therapists met with Sandra to develop a plan for the aftercare program. During the final treatment planning session, the results of the reevaluation were discussed and emphasis was given to resolving feelings regarding the major stressors of the past, ie. father's alcoholism, cancer and infertility. Encouragement was also given to pursue educational and career goals. Figure 9-11 contains the level three treatment plan. Sandra was given primary leadership in conducting the treatment planning meeting. Given the guideline that major issues of the addiction would be dealt with, Sandra indicated possible treatment goals and potential methods of reaching those goals.

The aftercare occupational therapist described some of the groups that were available in the aftercare program in order to facilitate Sandra's decision making regarding treatment strategies. Sandra and the aftercare occupational therapist scheduled individual sessions to discuss progress on goals. Time for the aftercare occupational therapist and Sandra to complete formal evaluations of progress were included in the treatment schedule as well.

Name _Sandra Jones_   **Date** _10/1/93_   **PDS Status** _3_

Functional Problems   Unresolved issues related to the addiction, deterioration of marital relationship, impoverishment of daily routine and limited number of roles.

Underlying Factors	**Strengths**
1. Lack of support system	1. Career goal (accountant)
2. Dependent on husband	2. Educational goal (obtain college degree)
3. Unresolved issues regarding father's drinking	3. Values marriage
4. Multiple stressors	4. Insight regarding stressors
	5. Able to keep scheduled appointments

Goals

LTG 3   By the end of one month, Sandra will remain abstinent with standby assist in order to improve the marital relationship.

> **STG 3a** Week two, Sandra will express with mod assist feelings related to father's drinking and other past stressors in order to remain abstinent.

> **STG 3b** Week three, Sandra will identify with min assist influence of father's drinking on current behaviors in order to remain abstinent.

> **STG 3c** Week four, Sandra will list with standby assist methods of altering influence of father's drinking on current behavior in order to remain abstinent.

LTG 4   By the end of one month, Sandra will independently add one new satisfying role to daily routine.

> **STG 4a** Week two, Sandra will institute with mod assist two interests into daily routine to fill gaps left by previous drinking.

> **STG 4b** Week three, Sandra will identify with min assist methods of meeting people.

> **STG 4c** Week four, Sandra will implement with standby assist two methods of meeting people.

Method   Issues Group 2 Xs/wk for one month and Role Identification Group 1 X/wk for one month.

Figure 9-11. Occupational therapy aftercare plan.

TREATMENT IMPLEMENTATION

One of the major differences between outpatient and inpatient treatment implementation relates to the fact that the substance abuser spends most of the time at home or on the job. It is therefore necessary for the substance abuser to complete much of the treatment independently in the discharge environment. Groups are conducted with this difference in mind. The substance abuser tries out new behaviors at home and then reports results back to the group members for additional feedback and encouragement. Group members are also given more freedom to conduct the group, directing topics to critical areas of emphasis. The aftercare occupational therapist has to deal with the often high dropout rate that can occur in outpatient substance abuse rehabilitation. As a result, the therapist maintains a critical eye on behaviors that indicate relapse. Relapse is a common occurrence that can be interrupted successfully without inpatient readmission if addressed promptly.

Sandra decided to attend the Issues Group two times per week and the Role Identification

Group one time per week for at least one month. The Issues group was a task group in which members selected activities that facilitated expression of unconscious conflicts. Sandra's goals emphasized resolution of issues related to her father's drinking, especially as it impacted her current role and performance functioning. The Issues group additionally utilized problem-solving strategies to facilitate the working through process. As a result, Sandra identified situations in which old feelings regarding her father were activated. Instead of responding with PDS behaviors as was true in the past during these situations, Sandra instituted healthy coping behaviors. Eventually the conflict lost its potency in terms of influencing behavior in a negative manner.

The Role Identification Group was designed to stimulate assumption of new roles. Sandra's goal was to add a new and challenging role to her routine that was in the past devoid of satisfying roles. Meaningful interests were added to her routine as well as methods of developing friendships.

FAMILY INVOLVEMENT

As in treatment level two, Mike's involvement in Sandra's aftercare occupational therapy program was important. Both the occupational therapist and Sandra agreed that it would not be appropriate for Mike to attend the Issues Group. In order for Sandra and other group members to freely experience and discuss unresolved feelings regarding past stressors, a comfortable and safe environment had to be provided. However, Mike needed to be aware of issues that affected the marital relationship. In this regard, indirect involvement in the occupational therapy aftercare program was warranted. Sandra used assertive communication to discuss her insights regarding old feelings and corresponding influence on behavior with her husband during marital therapy sessions and during time spent together at home.

Direct involvement of Mike in the Role Identification Group was possible. The occupational therapist held "open" group sessions in which family members shared observations about the substance abuser's successes in role performance and shared feedback regarding the impact on the family dynamics.

DISCHARGE PLANNING

Aftercare programs vary in length. Usually a month to two months is typical for most aftercare programs. Ideally, the substance abuser is monitored for a year to six months after discharge from the aftercare program. The occupational therapist based need for continued therapy on the goal progress discussion and from improvement measured by specific instruments. In fact, the occupational therapist made comparisons between pre- and post-testing of the Problem Situation Inventory.[8]

Results of the evaluation and the final goal progress discussion (conducted one month after initiation of the aftercare program) helped Sandra and the occupational therapist decide to discontinue the aftercare program. However, Sandra would meet with the occupational therapist in two months to explore readiness for implementation of educational goals and to assess Sandra's ability to maintain current level of functioning. Sandra and the occupational therapist also developed a home program that Sandra would follow in order to maintain current level of functioning. The home program consisted of keeping a daily diary to monitor stress and negative feelings, following a daily schedule that included newly developed interests and meeting with new social contacts, and implementing a variety of coping strategies to reduce stress levels and to dissipate negative emotions.

◆ CONCLUSIONS ◆

A hypothetical patient, generated from several composite cases treated by this author, was followed throughout the three hierarchical treatment levels. The example began with Sandra Jones being admitted to an inpatient drug and alcohol rehabilitation program. Upon receipt of referral, the occupational therapist initiated a chart review, an interview and a performance measure. Chart review indicated need for treatment level one approaches. The Occupational Case Analysis and Interview Rating Scale corroborated the conclusions made from the chart review as did the Comprehensive Occupational Therapy Evaluation Scale (COTE Scale).[1,2]

Tentative problems and strengths were synthesized from the data to formulate a treatment level one diagnosis. The problems relevant to treatment level one were presented to Sandra and pertinent goals were subsequently developed. Ways to measure progress were determined. From the diagnosis, the occupational therapist selected the model of human occupation to guide treatment. Ability to smoothly complete transition from one treatment level to another was a factor in selecting this frame of reference.

The COTE Scale monitored progress on basic task behaviors and interpersonal skills.[2] Spielberger's State-Trait Anxiety Scale assessed influence of biofeedback on reducing anxiety level.[3] These measurements, in conjunction with a discussion of goal progress, determined that Sandra was ready for treatment level two. The occupational therapy diagnosis was reformulated and a new treatment plan was developed . Additionally, specific methods to involve Sandra's husband in the occupational therapy program were delineated.

An assertiveness inventory, a coping skills assessment and a discussion of goal progress were used to determine readiness for treatment level three. The occupational therapist and the patient jointly met with the aftercare occupational therapist to develop an aftercare treatment plan. Change in treatment goals and methodology required an additional frame of reference. Two frames of reference were used because of the divergent nature of the two main treatment issues. Along with the usual discussion of goal progress, a measure of ability to handle relapse situations determined readiness for discharge from the aftercare program. A decision to discharge Sandra from the program was reached with agreement regarding number of necessary follow-up visits and need for a home program.

This case was ideal due to the lack of complications preventing goal progress. The case illustrated the way in which the three treatment levels guide clinical decision making. It is hoped that after reading and studying this case, the concepts inherent in the treatment levels are clearly understood and hold merit for clinical situations experienced by the reader.

References

1. Kaplan K, Kielhofner G: *Occupational Case Analysis Interview and Rating Scale.* Thorofare, NJ: Slack Inc., 1989.
2. Brayman SJ, Kirby TF, Misenheimer AM, Short MJ: Comprehensive occupational therapy evaluation scale. *Am J Occup Ther* 30: 94, 1976.
3. Spielberger CD, Gorsuch RI, Lushene RE: *Test Manual for the State-Trait Anxiety Inventory.* Palo Alto, CA: Consulting Psychologists Press, 1970.
4. Gambrill ED, Richey C: An assertion inventory for use in assessment and research. *Behav Res Ther* 6: 550-561, 1975.
5. Carver CS, Scheier MF, Weintraub JK: Assessing coping strategies: A theoretically based approach. *J Pers Soc Psychol* 56(2): 267-283, 1989.
6. Rotter JB: Generalized expectancies for internal vs. external control of reinforcement. *Psychology* Monogram 80 (Whole No. 609):1-28, 1966.
7. Beck AT: *Cognitive Therapy and Emotional Disorders.* New York: International Universities Press, 1976.
8. Hawkins JD, Catalano RF, Wells EA: Measuring effects of a skills training intervention for drug abusers. *J Consult Clin Psychol* 54(5): 661-664, 1986.

9. Lerner C, Ross G: The magazine picture collage: Development of an objective scoring system. *Am J Occup Ther* 31: 156-161, 1977.
10. Shostrom EL: *Personal Orientation Inventory (POI) Manual.* San Diego, CA: EDITS, 1974.
11. Holm M: Frames of reference: Guides for action. *Project for Independent Living in Occupational Therapy (PILOT).* Rockville, MD: American Occupational Therapy Association, 1986, pp. 69-78.

Trends in Substance Abuse
Rehabiliation

INTRODUCTION

In this chapter, current trends in the treatment of substance abuse are analyzed in terms of the potential impact upon occupational therapy. This chapter examines cost-effectiveness of substance abuse treatment and the corresponding funding issues. Conducting treatment efficacy research in order to enhance reimbursement of services for the substance abuser is advocated.

◆ COST-EFFECTIVENESS ◆

Within the substance abuse literature, there is substantial evidence supporting the cost-benefit of treatment. Jones and Vischi reviewed the treatment benefits of substance abuse programs over a ten-year period.[1] Each of the studies evaluated by Jones and Vischi found that substance abuse treatment produced reductions in medical care utilization and corresponding expenditures.[1] In fact, the median reduction in sick days and accident benefits was 40 percent.[1] Based on cost-benefit research, the positive effects of substance abuse treatment outweigh the costs of providing treatment.[2-7]

Probably one of the more influential cost-benefit analyses was conducted by Holder, Blose and Basiorowski.[8] This study examined the impact of substance abuse treatment on overall health care utilization and costs for individuals and families filing claims with Aetna Life Insurance Company under the Federal Employees Health Benefit Program. From this data, it was determined that families, with at least one member filing a claim for substance abuse treatment during 1980-1983, used health care services and incurred costs at a rate about twice that of a comparison group.

Additionally, it was reported that a gradual rise in overall health care costs and health care use occurred for substance abusers during the three years preceding substance abuse treatment.[8] In fact, the most dramatic increase in costs and health care use seemed to occur in the six months prior to treatment for substance abuse. Consequently, after the substance abusers received treatment for the substance abuse, their general health care costs dropped dramatically and eventually reached approximately the level that existed several years prior to substance abuse treatment.[8] Using a variety of forecasting techniques, the average substance abuser's treatment cost was offset by reductions in other health care costs within approximately two to three years following the start of substance abuse treatment.[8]

Many substance abuse treatment services, however, are not cost-effective. There are probably less expensive ways of providing treatment than are currently reflected in reimbursement policy.[9] Medicare and Medicaid, for instance, emphasize the most expensive treatment services, ie. inpatient, medically-based treatment. Currently, third party payers are questioning the wisdom of this policy and are searching for cost-effective treatment methods that produce the most cost-benefits.

This search for cost-effective treatment is heightened by the continuing demand for employers to provide substance-abuse treatment. As a result, some businesses are using independent Employee Assistance Programs (EAPs) that employ social workers and psychologists rather than psychiatrists as a cost savings measure to inpatient treatment.[10] In general, supporting employees through treatment for substance abuse is cost-effective.[11] A McDonnell Douglas study, described by Castelli, suggested that the EAP produced a savings of four dollars for every dollar spent by the program.[11] Also according to Castelli, the Hillsborough Area Regional Transit in Tampa had $1,013,209 in liability costs for personal and property damage in 1984. After implementing an extensive EAP program that addressed the substance abuse of the employees, the same costs had dropped to $29,951 by 1986.

◆ FUNDING ISSUES ◆

During the 1980s, private insurance companies, employers and the federal government expanded benefits for substance abuse treatment. As a result of expanded benefits during this time period, the number of inpatient psychiatric beds treating substance-abuse patients increased by 50 percent.[10] In fact, chemical-dependency treatment costs jumped 53 percent during the period between 1986-1987.[10] A Bureau of Labor Statistics 1985 survey of over 1300 health insurance plans offered by medium-sized and large firms found that 68 percent of all participants had some coverage for the treatment of substance abuse.[10] This figure was up from 38 percent in 1981 and from 61 percent in 1984. In fact, 36 states as of 1985 required some form of substance abuse coverage in health insurance policies sold in their states.[12]

With the advent of escalating health-care costs, the major issue is whether current reimbursement policies support the provision of the most cost-effective treatment.[13] In the late 1980s up through the 1990s, cost containment has wielded its influence upon the way in which substance abusers receive treatment. The traditional 28-day inpatient treatment programs have been shortened to a time period between 17 and 22 days.[14] Many of the Health Maintenance Organizations (HMO) limit inpatient coverage to two to three days, supposedly covering the detoxification period.[9] Treatment is moving to the outpatient setting. However, outpatient mental health benefits are not consistently included in the health insurance policies of individuals. In general, nonhospital based treatment programs, including outpatient care, aftercare and nonmedically oriented residential care, are less frequently reimbursed by private insurance companies and by governmental insurance programs.

GOVERNMENT INSURANCE PROGRAMS

The major payers of substance abuse treatment services, remain the federal, state and local governmental agencies. As of October, 1987, alcohol and substance abuse inpatient facilities were included in the prospective payment system (PPS) of Medicare.[13] Prior to 1987, the Department of Health and Human Services gave alcohol and substance abuse facilities the option of remaining exempt from PPS. The DRG (Diagnostic Related Group) rates for substance abuse are criticized as being too low for the current level of treatment. These complaints arise from that fact that HCFA (Health Care Financing Administration) included the costs of less specialized providers in its DRG calculations.[13]

Outcome studies questioning the effectiveness of inpatient treatment are being used to justify cuts in payment for inpatient treatment.[15] While a report on the impact of a prospective payment method supports the notion that preset levels of reimbursement reduce hospitalization costs for mental health medicare patients, cost reductions are possibly offset by higher readmission rates or charges.[16] As a result, prospective reimbursement schemes may not have an impact on the total cost of mental health care over a period of time. Instead, prospective reimbursement has a greater influence on changing the pattern of care.

In actuality though, the effect of Medicare's cost controls upon substance abuse treatment facilities may be minimal due to the low percentages of Medicare patients receiving treatment for substance abuse. Only four to five percent of the revenue for certain private treatment facilities is generated from Medicare patients.[13] In fact, payments to substance-abuse treatment facilities are a small part of the government's health budget, ie. $53.1 million in 1987 or about one percent of HCFA's $45 billion in payments to hospitals.[13]

The hospital industry is currently looking to the Defense Department as an indicator of what other payers will do to control costs of substance abuse and drug rehabilitation.[13] Hospitals authorized to treat the 6.2 million beneficiaries of CHAMPUS (the Civilian Health and Medical Program of the Uniformed Services) are paid according to Medicare DRG rates. However, substance abuse rehabilitation facilities are exempt from the CHAMPUS prospective payment program. Currently, CHAMPUS is studying alternative approaches to pay for these services. The reason for the influence of CHAMPUS upon other payers of substance abuse rehabilitation relates to the fact that CHAMPUS covers patients of all ages. Medicare, in contrast, is primarily restricted to the 65 and older age group. Therefore, it is felt by the insurance industry that CHAMPUS better reflects the patient groups covered by other payers.[13]

The medicaid program (Title XIX of the Social Security Act) is funded by the federal government and by individual states for the purpose of providing medical assistance to persons with low incomes. States have substantial leeway in administering the program as long as certain basic health services are provided. For instance, Medicaid state plans must include inpatient psychiatric services for individuals less than 21 years of age and for individuals more than 65 years of age. Outpatient services that include Community Mental Health Centers, clinics, outpatient hospitals, and other alternatives to public institutional care are also required for these individuals.[14]

The Medicaid program excludes federal financial participation for the care of persons between the ages of 21 and 65 in psychiatric institutions.[17] This limitation excludes those low income persons, between the ages of 21 and 65, from receiving inpatient substance abuse treatment unless other provisions are made by state governments. However, Medicaid statutes fail to specifically mention provisions for substance abuse treatment for all age groups. According to Ferguson and Kirk, Medicaid provided six percent ($5 million) of the total funds to NIAAA-funded substance abuse treatment centers.[18] In general though, most state Medicaid agencies fail to reimburse for treatment of substance abuse unless it is provided in a medical setting.[19]

OTHER PAYERS

Coverage for psychiatric services in general and for substance-abuse treatment specifically by private insurance is inconsistent. Traditionally, mental health benefits have limitations in the form of caps on total coverage available, higher coinsurance and larger deductibles. These limitations are more restrictive than the general medical coverages offered.[20]

Some private insurance companies have adopted payment systems similar to Medicare's prospective payment program. Blue Cross of Arizona, for example, has paid for substance-abuse treatment using Medicare's DRGs since their implementation in 1983.[13] The application of Medicare DRGs may be inappropriate due to the fact that differences are not accounted for between the treatment population and the Medicare population. To illustrate this problem, consider the fact that an adolescent's average hospital stay for substance-abuse treatment is 30 to 35 days as compared to the Medicare patient's average stay of 16 to 17 days.[13]

In terms of funding, managed care insurance plans (eg. health maintenance organizations [HMOs] and preferred provider organizations [PPOs]) have produced the greatest impact upon substance abuse and psychiatric hospitals. These funding programs are popular as a consequence of employers demanding less costly health insurance alternatives. Managed care programs (HMOs and PPOs) typically negotiate with treatment providers reduced service rates. Emphasis is placed upon providing, when possible, less-intensive treatment settings.

Managed care is also characterized by strong utilization review components that require preadmission certification as a method of restricting the numbers of costly inpatient admissions and determining appropriateness of health care service utilization. Insurance industry surveys show that 75 percent of all inpatient psychiatric admissions are subject to prior approval.[10] Many prepaid plans (HMOs) permit only a short two- or three-day hospitalization when the average is usually 12 days for most psychiatric diagnoses.[10]

◆ IMPACT ON OCCUPATIONAL THERAPY ◆

RESEARCH

Specific trends in the substance abuse rehabilitation field impact occupational therapy. Funding for the inpatient treatment of substance abuse in the early 1980s steadily increased, but now funding seems to be in jeopardy. Decreased funding is occurring despite the fact that treatment costs are offset by a reduction in general health-care costs once the substance abuser receives treatment for the addiction. Rising health-care costs have forced employers and the insurance industry to determine more cost-effective treatment so that cost-benefits can be realized. It is expected that insurance companies and employers in the future will demand proof of treatment effectiveness and cost-benefit. Insurance companies are interested in those treatment approaches that can be administered on an outpatient basis and that require the services of less expensive personnel.

These key points raise several issues. Occupational therapists must conduct treatment effectiveness and cost-benefit studies, analyzing the outcomes attributable to occupational therapy intervention. The occupational therapy literature contains few research studies determining the benefits of intervention. The occupational therapy treatment approach described in this book requires validation through research. A theoretical foundation as a guide to practice and to research has been provided, but this foundation is not enough in terms of satisfying third party payers.

A treatment service that can produce data substantiating effectiveness, both in terms of outcomes and in terms of cost savings, is well ahead of other mental health professions. This data enhances funding and ensures that substance abusers have access to the treatment they need in order to recover. Services that fail to substantiate claims of positive outcomes will not be funded in the future.

Involvement of occupational therapists in the treatment of substance abusers has potential to increase. Research indicates that treatment for substance abuse is successful in achieving cessation or reduction of addictive behaviors over the short run, but maintaining these positive changes over time is less likely to occur.[21] Current treatment does not substantially influence the life context and coping factors that are closely linked to the process of remission and relapse. The findings of Moos, Finney and Cronkite indicate that treatment should be oriented toward strengthening natural recovery processes and improving the life contexts of patients and their ability to manage these contexts.[22] The functional treatment methods advocated by this book address both these necessary factors for long-term treatment effectiveness.

DOCUMENTATION

Even more basic than treatment effectiveness research is illustrating the contributions to substance abuse rehabilitation through appropriate documentation of patient care. Documentation that enhances reimbursement incorporates the standards set forth in the Medicare Part B Occupational Therapy Guidelines.[23] Regardless of payment source, utilizing these guidelines is important. Medicare Part B Guidelines are the only official description of the documentation process. The guidelines clearly define "skilled" occupational therapy and the components of a reimbursable service. For example, evaluating the patient's current functional abilities is a skilled service. Teaching assertiveness skills without having the patient apply the techniques is a nonskilled occupational therapy service.

Figure 10-1 reviews the basic patient-care documentation principles set forth in the Medicare Part B Guidelines.[23] Note the emphasis upon documenting the patient's baseline functional performance, determining the rehabilitation potential, setting long-term functional goals, delineating the duration and frequency of treatment, analyzing the underlying factors contributing to functional performance deficits, providing skilled occupational therapy, and describing the patient's response to treatment.

Proper documentation clearly delineates occupational therapy from other services provided by social workers, psychologists or recreational therapists. Avoiding unnecessary duplication of other services is necessary in order to enhance cost-benefits. Secondly, functional outcomes are predicted and specific "skilled" methods are designed to produce desired outcomes suggestive

Table 10-1
Essential Aspects

Medicare Part-B (1989) Guidelines

I. Patient history
 A. Determine prior level of functioning
 B. Medical history
  1. Treatment diagnosis
  2. Date of onset
  3. Date of exacerbation
  4. Dates of medical procedures
 C. Occupational therapy history

II. Technical review items
 A. Facility and patient identification
 B. Physician referral
  1. Receipt of referral date
  2. Referral source
  3. Referral purpose
 C. Date of last certification, if applicable
 D. Number of visits, if applicable
 E. Date treatment started (date OT was initiated)
 F. Billing period

III. Evaluation
 A. Use standardized evaluations when possible
 B. Evaluate functional abilities and limitations
 C. Determine underlying factors
 D. Assess rehabilitation potential

IV. Treatment plan
 A. Develop reasonable goals
 B. Delineate functional goals (long-term goals)
  1. Incorporate assistance levels
   a. Total assistance
   b. Maximum assistance
   c. Moderate assistance
   d. Minimum assistance
   e. Standby assistance
   f. Independent
  2. Or incorporate changes within assistance levels
   a. Decreased refusals
   b. Increased consistency
   c. Increased generalization
   d. A new functional skill is initiated
   e. Added new skilled compensatory technique
   f. Increased time treatment is tolerated
  3. Functional goal content
   a. ADL (not limited to the following:)
    1) Feed, eat, drink
    2) Bathe
    3) Dress
    4) Perform personal hygiene
    5) Groom
    6) Perform toileting

Table 10-1
Essential Aspects

      b. Safety (not limited to the following:)
         1) High probability of falling
         2) Lack of environmental safety awareness
         3) Swallowing difficulties
         4) Aggressive/destructive behavior
         5) Severe pain
         6) Loss of skin sensation
         7) Progressive joint contracture
         8) Need for joint protection/preservation
      c. Input from patient and/or caregiver

C. Delineate goals that remediate underlying factors (not limited to the following:)
    1. Lacks awareness of sensory cues or safety hazards
    2. Impaired attention span
    3. Impaired strength
    4. Incoordination
    5. Abnormal muscle tone
    6. Range of motion limitations
    7. Impaired body scheme
    8. Perceptual deficits
    9. Impaired balance/head control
    10. Environmental barriers

D. Select specific treatment methods
    1. Skilled occupational therapy
      a. Evaluation
      b. Determining services in conjunction with the patient/caregiver
      c. Analyzing and modifying functional tasks
      d. Determining optimal level of performance for a task
      e. Providing instructions to the patient/caregivers
      f. Periodic reevaluation
    2. Avoid unskilled occupational therapy
      a. Maintenance
      b. Continuing therapy even no progress
      c. Duplicating services of other professionals
      d. Routine practice
      e. Skill education without practice
      f. Routine strengthening or exercise

E. Specify frequency and duration of treatment

V. Progress reporting
  A. Progress on functional goals
    1. Change in assistance levels
    2. Change within assistance levels
  B. Type of skilled services implemented
  C. Response to skilled services
  D. Modify treatment plan

Table 10-1
Essential Aspects

Medicare Part-B (1989) Guidelines (continued)

VI. Discharge
    A. Discontinue when skilled services no longer indicated
    B. Specify actual functional outcomes
    C. Summarize treatment implemented
    D. Develop and train regarding home program
    E. Delineate criteria for future referral

---

of quality health care. Insurance companies and employers are interested in functional behaviors that decrease the likelihood of relapse and treatment recidivism.

Functionally-based documentation deemphasizes performance components, ie. cognitive, social, sensorimotor and psychological skills. Underlying factors contributing to or limiting function are addressed in treatment. The connection, however, between performance components and function is clearly described. For example, it is not enough to document that a substance abuser has cognitive deficits related to memory impairment and problem solving difficulties. The effect that these cognitive deficits have upon occupational performances must be clear, eg. because of short-term memory loss, the substance abuser requires maximum assistance in order to follow a daily schedule.

Documentation also describes how the occupational therapist skillfully augments the substance abuser's short-term memory through training care-givers in the use of memory aids. Modification of the environment enables the substance abuser to follow a daily schedule with less assistance.

SITE OF SERVICE DELIVERY

Another major implication for occupational therapy is the site of service delivery. As stated, employers and insurance companies are aware of the high costs associated with inpatient substance abuse treatment programs. The cost-effectiveness literature indicates that outpatient programs are as clinically effective as inpatient treatment programs and are less expensive as well. Based on these results, reimbursement policy is directing funds to outpatient sites of treatment delivery for certain substance abusers. As a result, occupational therapists must design services conducive to outpatient, aftercare, and to employee assistant programs. It will be detrimental for the occupational therapy program to be exclusively connected with inpatient services.

PAYMENT

Occupational therapists must consider the perspective of insurance companies and employers when deciding whether to bill for occupational therapy services or to include the cost as a part of a program treatment cost, eg. including inpatient occupational therapy within the per diem or outpatient occupational therapy within the total program costs. There are problems and advantages to both billing methodologies.

Cost containment efforts by third party payers, in some cases, dictate the billing methodology. This is certainly true of Medicare. Medicare pays a prospective flat rate for the diagnostic category regardless of the actual inpatient treatment costs. Generally, the type of services provided the Medicare patient are left up to the inpatient facility as long as utilization review indicates that the standard treatment approaches were implemented. Managed care programs or preferred provider organizations may also negotiate a flat rate with the substance abuse inpatient or outpatient treatment facility for the total program. Fee for service may eventually become an outmoded method of billing.

If occupational therapy is included as part of a program treatment fee, the occupational therapist needs to maintain or increase the visibility of the service. Public relations materials that include descriptions of the occupational therapy program could help influence employers or insurance companies to select the substance abuse rehabilitation facility as its "preferred provider." In the case of Medicare DRGs, it is important for the occupational therapy program to document impact upon speed of recovery so that transfer to a less expensive type of care (aftercare) can occur before the hospital costs exceed the prospective rate. The advantage of being included as a part of a global treatment rate involves the ability for all patients in the facility to receive the necessary occupational therapy services. The occupational therapist does not have to be as careful to limit services to those minimally necessary as might be the case when billing each session separately.

The advantage of billing for occupational therapy services, whether inpatient or outpatient, relates to the visibility afforded the service. Occupational therapy is viewed as a profit center by administrators. Often this viewpoint provides increased power to the occupational therapy department in terms of budget control, program planning and development and hiring of staff. Disadvantages result from the lack of inclusion of occupational therapy as a mental health benefit in many private insurance policies. Participation in the occupational therapy program by substance abusers devoid of the appropriate insurance coverage may, as a result, be limited. It is important for occupational therapists to develop plans to improve reimbursement coverage by the majority of the treatment population's insurance programs.

The occupational therapy program manager needs to monitor, additionally, any changes in coverage implemented by the major third party payers for the patient population. The manager needs to be cognizant of the relationship between amount billed versus actual reimbursement received for services. Denials of coverage require investigation and, in some cases, appeal of the decision. Patient documentation is crucial to avoid denials of payment and to demonstrate the appropriateness and effectiveness of the service in obtaining desired functional outcomes.

PREVENTION

The pressure to reduce health care spending will continue. Cost containment raises the issue of a two-tiered health-care system. Searching for methods to pay for indigent health-care and to maintain access to a basic level of services is imperative. There has been a steady decline in the numbers of public inebriate programs.[24] In terms of cost-benefits, prevention is a cheaper alternative to treatment of substance abuse. As of yet, occupational therapists have not developed a role in substance abuse prevention programs. This is an area that deserves exploration, especially given the current funding environment.

Particularly promising is the prevention approach that emphasizes education for responsible decision-making.[25] This approach is based upon the understanding that personal attitudes toward responsible behavior are first developed within the family setting. Research indicates that parents teach norms regarding the use of alcohol and other drugs. These norms are influential in an individual's future drug use pattern.[26,27] Consequently, parents have a responsibility for reexamining their own values before knowingly or unknowingly imposing them upon their children.

This particular prevention strategy works with parents to incorporate into their value systems the following values regarding responsible behavior: 1) it is not essential to use drugs; 2) uncontrolled drug use is a health problem; 3) drugs are dangerous when used to solve emotional problems; 4) drunkenness or artificially altered emotional and cognitive states are not to be tolerated and are socially unacceptable; and 5) drug education is actually only one aspect of learning to cope with life problems.[25] Occupational therapists are qualified to develop and implement life coping training programs that involve parents and their children.

◆ CONCLUSIONS ◆

This chapter examined the future of substance abuse treatment and the resulting impact upon occupational therapy. Of grave concern is the effect of continuing, aggressive cost containment upon the future of substance abuse treatment. Generally, the costs of not treating substance abuse far outweigh the costs associated with treatment. Reimbursement policies are being reexamined in terms of changing the emphasis upon inpatient treatment in favor of alternative, less costly treatment approaches. As a result, it is necessary for occupational therapists to develop programming that meets the needs of substance abusers treated on an outpatient basis.

Research by occupational therapists examining the impact of intervention upon functional outcomes is important. The funding environment emphasizes quality of care. Insurance programs and employers are interested in providing the most effective treatment at a given cost. Occupational therapists not only need to provide data indicating the effectiveness of treatment, but need to illustrate the cost-benefits of the service. To substantiate the research effort, occupational therapists must incorporate functionally-based patient documentation into current documentation procedures. This documentation communicates the importance of occupational therapy to the substance abuser's recovery process.

Monitoring changes in funding methodology is necessary to maintain appropriate billing strategies for the occupational therapy service. Fee-for-service billing will eventually be obsolete, especially given that Medicare has implemented cost controls for ambulatory and physician fees. Other private insurers will likely adopt similar cost containment methods. Consequently, occupational therapy programs must demonstrate significant contributions to improved treatment outcomes.

Involvement in prevention programs may compensate for the high cost of treatment. Rather than waiting for the person to become a substance abuser and then providing services, the hope is to stop the individual from developing substance abuse in the first place. Helping parents to reexamine values that may possibly contribute to the unwitting acceptance by their children of drug usage in times of stress could be the focus of such prevention efforts.

The purpose of this book was to help occupational therapists resolve problems in the treatment of substance abuse. This book provides a framework for treatment that differentiates occupational therapy from other mental health services, produces specific functional outcomes, delineates intervention approaches and stimulates research in the field of substance abuse. The primary goal here is to encourage occupational therapists to increase their involvement in the treatment of substance abuse. It is a health problem that will continue to have broad impact on society in general for decades in the future.

References

1. Jones KR, Vischi TR: *Impact of alcohol drug abuse, and mental health treatment on medical care utilization: A review of the research literature.* Med Care 17 (Supplement), 1979.
2. Brock CB, Boyaty TG: *Group Health Association of America Study: Alcoholism within Prepaid Group Practice HMOs* (Report to NIAAA No. 5HAA01745). Washington, DC: U.S. Government Printing Office, 1978.
3. Sherman RM, Reiff S, Forsythe AB: Utilization of medical services by alcoholics participating in an outpatient treatment program. *Alcohol Clin Exp Res 3(115), 1979.*
4. Hunter H: *Arizona Health Plan Cost-benefit Study* (Report to NIAAA No. 5h84AA01745). Washington, DC: U.S. Government Printing Office, 1978.
5. Hayami DE, Freebori DK: Effect of coverage in the use of HMO alcoholism treatment program, outcome and medical care utilization. *Am J Pub Health* 71: 1133-1144, 1981.
6. Holder HD, Hallan JB: *The California Pilot Program to Provide Health Insurance Coverage for Alcohol Treatment—One Year After.* Chapel Hill, NC: H-2, Inc., 1978.
7. Holder HD, Hallan JB: *Medical Care and Alcoholism Treatment Costs and Utilization: A Five-year Analysis of the California Pilot Project to Provide Health Insurance Coverage for Alcoholism.* Chapel Hill, NC: H-2, Inc., 1981.
8. Holder HD, Blose JG, Basiorowski MH: *Alcoholism Treatment Impact on Total Health Care Utilization and Costs: A Four-year Longitudinal Analysis of the Federal Employees Health Benefit Program with AETNA Life Insurance Program.* Chapel Hill, NC: H-2, Inc., 1985.
9. Saxe L, Dougherty D, Esty K: The effectiveness and cost of alcoholism treatment: A public policy perspective. In Mendelson JH & Mello NK (Eds.): *The Diagnosis and Treatment of Alcoholism.* New York: McGraw-Hill, 1985, pp. 485-540.
10. Robinson ML: Psych: PPS may be out, but the pressure is on. *Hospitals* June 5: 28-30, 1989.
11. Castelli J: Addiction employer-provided programs pay off. *HR Mag* April: 55-58, 1990.
12. Korcok M: Alcoholism treatment a growing "product line." *Am Med News* October 11: 29-30, 1985.
13. Wallace C: Specialty providers fear PPS. *Modern Healthcare* January 15: 20-21, 28, 30, 1988.
14. Peters ME: Reimbursement for psychiatric occupational therapy services. *Am J Occup Ther* 38(5): 307-312, 1984.
15. Mezochow J, Miller S, Seixas F, Frances RJ: The impact of cost containment on alcohol and drug treatment. *Hosp Com Psych* 38(5): 506-510, 1987.
16. Rupp A, Steinwachs DM, Salkever DS: The effect of hospital payment methods on the pattern and cost of mental health care. *Hos Com Psych* 35: 456-459, 1984.
17. *National Institute of Alcohol Abuse and Alcoholism, Information and Feature Service*: AA Survey Reflects More Diverse Membership (IFS No. 91) December 31. Rockville, MD: Author, 1981.
18. Ferguson L, Kirk J: *Statistical Report: National Institute on Alcohol Abuse and Alcoholism-funded Treatment Programs, Calendar Year 1978.* Rockville, MD: National Institute on Alcohol Abuse and Alcoholism, Alcohol, Drug Abuse and Mental Health Administration, 1979.
19. *Health Care Financing Administration: Coverage of Alcoholism Treatment Services Titles XVIII and XIX*, August 24, 1979. Department of Health, Education, and Welfare, Washington, DC, 1979.
20. Williams SJ, Torrens PR: *Introduction to Health Services* (3rd ed.). New York: John Wiley & Sons, 1988.
21. Maisto SA, Sobell LC, Sobell MB, Sanders B: Effects of outpatient treatment for problem drinkers. *Am J Drug Alcohol Abuse* 11: 131-149, 1985.
22. Moos RH, Finney JW, Cronkite RC: *Alcoholism Treatment Context, Process, and Outcome.* New York: Oxford University Press, 1990.
23. *Health Care Financing Administration: Medicare Outpatient Physical Therapy and Comprehensive Outpatient Rehabilitation Facility Manual.* Washington DC: Author, Transmittal No. 87:98-111a, 1989.
24. Yahr HT: A national comparison of public- and private-sector alcoholism treatment delivery system characteristics. *J Stud Alcohol* 49(3): 233-239, 1988.
25. Chafetz M, Yoerg R: Public health treatment programs in alcoholism. In Kissin B, Begleiter H (Eds.): *The Biology of Alcoholism* Vol 5: Treatment and Rehabilitation of the Chronic Alcoholic. New York: Plenum Press, pp. 593-614, 1977.
26. Barnes GM: The development of adolescent drinking behaviors: An evaluative review of the impact of the socialization process within the family. *Adolescence* 12: 571-591, 1977.
27. McDermott D: The relationship of parental drug use and parents' attitude concerning adolescent drug use to adolescent drug use. *Adolescence* 19: 89-97, 1984.

Resources

◆ FRAMES OF REFERENCE ◆

Overview of Frames of Reference Used in Occupational Therapy

Bruce MA, Borg B: *Frames of Reference in Psychosocial Occupational Therapy.* Thorofare, NJ: Slack Inc., 1987.

Robertson SC (Ed.): *FOCUS: Skills for Assessment and Treatment.* Rockville, MD: The American Occupational Therapy Association, Inc., 1988.

Management of Cognitive Disabilities

Allen, CK: *Occupational Therapy for Psychiatric Diseases: Measurement and Management of Cognitive Disabilities.* Boston, MA: Little, Brown, 1985.

Action Consequence

Mosey AC: *Psychosocial Components of Occupational Therapy.* New York: Raven Press, 1986.

Model of Human Occupation

Kielhofner G (Ed): *A Model of Human Occupation: Theory and Application.* Baltimore, MD: Williams and Wilkins, 1985.

Cognitive-Behavioral

Bruce MA, Borg B: *Frames of Reference in Psychosocial Occupational Therapy.* Thorofare, NJ: Slack Inc., 1987.

Meichenbaum D: *Cognitive-behavior Modification.* New York: Plenum Press, 1977.

Ellis A: *Reason and Emotion in Psychotherapy.* New York: Lyle Stuart, 1962.

Emery G, Hollon SD, Bedrosian RC: *New Directions in Cognitive Therapy: A Casebook.* New York: The Guilford Press, 1981.

Object Relations

Mosey AC: *Three Frames of Reference for Mental Health.* Thorofare, NJ: Slack Inc., 1970.

Mosey AC: *Psychosocial Components of Occupational Therapy.* New York: Raven Press, 1986.

◆ TREATMENT LEVEL ONE EVALUATIONS ◆

COGNITIVE

Allen Cognitive Level (ACL): Lower Cognitive Level (LCL)

Allen, CK: *Occupational Therapy for Psychiatric Diseases: Measurement and Management of Cognitive Disabilities.* Boston, MA: Little Brown, 1985.

Allen Cognitive Level: Problem-Solving Version (ACL-PS)

Josman N, Katz N: A problem-solving version of the Allen Cognitive Level Test. *AJOT* 45(4): 331-339.

Loewenstein Occupational Therapy Cognitive Assessment

Itzkovich M, Elazar B, Aberbuch S: *Loewenstein Occupational Therapy Cognitive Assessment (LOTCA) Manual.* Pequannock, NJ: Maddak, Inc., 1990.

Bay Area Functional Performance Evaluation: Task-Oriented Assessment (BaFPE-TOA)

Bloomer J, Williams S: The Bay Area Functional Performance Evaluation. In Hemphill B (Ed.): *The Evaluative Process in Psychiatric Occupational Therapy.* Thorofare, NJ: Slack Inc., 1982, pp. 255-308.

Test Publisher
Consulting Psychologists Press, Inc.
577 College Ave.
Palo Alto, CA 94306

Cognitive Adaptive Skills Evaluation (CASE)

Masagatani GN, Nielson CS, Ranslow ER: *Cognitive Adaptive Skills Evaluation Manual.* New York: Haworth Press, 1981.

Elizur Test of Psycho-organicity

Elizur, A: *ETPO Test Administration Booklet*. Los Angeles: Western Psychological Service, 1969.

Test Publisher
Western Psychological Service
12031 Wilshire Boulevard
Los Angeles, CA 90025

Quick Neurological Screening Test (QNST)

Mutti M, Sterling HM, Spalding NV: *Quick Neurological Screening Test* (Rev. ed). Novato, CA: Academic Therapy Publications, 1978.

Test Publisher
Western Psychological Service
12031 Wilshire Boulevard
Los Angeles, CA 90025

Dynamic Investigation

Toglia JP: Approaches to cognitive assessment of the brain-injured adult: Traditional methods and dynamic investigation. *Occup Ther Practice* 1(1): 36-57, 1989a.

Toglia JP: Visual perception of objects: An approach to assessment and intervention. *AJOT* 43(9): 589-595, 1989b.

PSYCHOLOGICAL

State-Trait Anxiety Inventory

Spielberger CD: *Manual for the State-Trait Anxiety Inventory*. Palo Alto, CA: Consulting Psychologists Press, 1983.

Test Publisher
Consulting Psychologists Press, Inc.
577 College Ave.
Palo Alto, CA 94306

IPAT Anxiety Scale Questionnaire (Self-Analysis Form)

Krug SE: *Handbook for IPAT Anxiety Scale*. Champaign, IL: Institute for Personality and Ability Testing, 1976.

Test Publisher
Western Psychological Service
12031 Wilshire Boulevard
Los Angeles, CA 90025

Internal/External Scale

Rotter JB: Generalized expectancies for internal versus external control of reinforcement. *Psych Mon* 80: 1-28, 1966.

Hopelessness Scale

Beck AT, Weissman A, Lester D, Prexler L: The measurement of pessimism: The Hopelessness Scale. *J Consul Clin Psych* 42: 867-865, 1974.

Tennessee Self-Concept Scale

Fitts WH: *Manual: Tennessee Self-Concept Scale.* Los Angeles: Western Psychological Services, 1965.

Test Publisher
Western Psychological Service
12031 Wilshire Boulevard
Los Angeles, CA 90025

Self-Esteem Scale

Rosenberg M: *Society and the Adolescent Self-image.* Princeton, NJ: Princeton University Press, 1965.

Robinson J, Shaver, P: *Measures of Social Psychological Attitudes.* Ann Arbor, MI: Institute of Social Research, 1973, pp. 81-83.

SOCIAL

Bay Area Functional Performance Evaluation—Social Interaction Scale (BaFPE-SIS)

Bloomer J, Williams S: The Bay Area Functional Performance Evaluation. In Hemphill B (Ed.): *The Evaluative Process in Psychiatric Occupational Therapy.* Thorofare, NJ: Slack Inc., 1982, pp. 255-308.

Test Publisher
Consulting Psychologists Press, Inc.
577 College Ave.
Palo Alto, CA 94306

Comprehensive Occupational Therapy Evaluation (COTE)

Brayman SJ, Kirby T: Comprehensive occupational therapy evaluation. *AJOT* 30(2): 94-100.

Occupational Case Analysis Interview and Rating Scale (OCAIRS)

Kaplan KL, Kielhofner G: *Occupational Case Analysis Interview and Rating Scale.* Thorofare, NJ: Slack Inc., 1989.

Test Publisher
Slack Inc.
6900 Grove Road
Thorofare, NJ 08086

SENSORIMOTOR

SBC Adult Psychiatric Sensory Integration Evaluation (SBC)

Van Schroeder, Block MP, Trottier EC, Stowell MS: *SBC Adult Psychiatric Sensory Integration Evaluation.* Kailua, HA: Schroeder Publishing and Consulting, 1983.

Person Symbol

Hemphill, B (Ed): *The Evaluative Process in Psychiatric Occupational Therapy.* Thorofare, NJ: Slack Inc., 1982.

Developmental Test of Visual-Motor Integration (VMI)

Beery KE, Buktenica NA: *Developmental Test of Visual-motor Integration.* Cleveland, OH: Modern Curriculum Press, 1982.

Hooper Visual Organization Chart (VOT)

Hooper HE: *Hooper Visual Organization Chart.* Los Angeles: Western Psychological Services, 1983.

Test Publisher
Western Psychological Services
12031 Wilshire Boulevard
Los Angeles, CA 90025

Minnesota Spatial Relations Test (MSRT)

Davis, RV: *Minnesota Spatial Relations Test (MSRT).* Circle Pines, MN: American Guidance Service, 1979.

Test Publisher
American Guidance Service, Inc.
Publishers Building
Circle Pines, MN 55014

Motor-Free Visual Perception Test (MVPT)

Bouska MJ, Kwatny E: *Motor-free Visual Perception Test (MVPT).* Novato, CA: Academic Therapy Publications, 1983.

Test Publisher
Academic Therapy Publications
20 Commercial Blvd.
Novato, CA 94947-6191

Purdue Pegboard

Tiffin J: *Purdue Pegboard Examiner Manual.* Chicago, IL: Science Research Associates, 1986.

Test Publisher
Lafayette Instrument Company
Sagamore Parkway & 9th Street
Lafayette, IN 47903

ACTIVITIES OF DAILY LIVING

Routine Task Inventory/Routine Task History Interview

Allen, CK: *Occupational Therapy for Psychiatric Diseases: Measurement and Management of Cognitive Disabilities.* Boston, MA: Little Brown, 1985.

Comprehensive Evaluation of Basic Living Skills (CEBLS)

Casanova JS, Ferber J: Comprehensive evaluation of basic living skills. *AJOT* 30: 101-105, 1976.

Kohlman Evaluation of Living Skills (KELS)

Thomson, LK: *Kohlman evaluation of daily living skills (KELS).* Rockland, MD: AOTA, 1992.

Test Publisher
American Occupational Therapy Association
1383 Piccard Drive
PO Box 1725
Rockville, MD 20849-1725

The Scorable Self-Care Evaluation (SSCE)

Peters, M, Clark, N: *Scorable Self-care Evaluation.* Thorofare, NJ: Slack Inc., 1984.

Test Publisher
Slack Inc.
6900 Grove Road
Thorofare, NJ 08086

The Milwaukee Evaluation of Daily Living Skills (MEDLS)

Leonardelli CA: *The Milwaukee Evaluation of Daily Living Skills: Evaluation in Long-term Psychiatric Care.* Thorofare, NJ: Slack Inc., 1988.

Test Publisher
Slack Inc.
6900 Grove Road
Thorofare, NJ 08086

Activity Configuration

Mosey A: *Activities Therapy.* New York: Raven Press, 1973.

Hemphill B (Ed): *The Evaluative Process in Psychiatric Occupational Therapy.* Thorofare, NJ: Slack Inc., 1988.

Barth Time Construction

Hemphill B (Ed): *The Evaluative Process in Psychiatric Occupational Therapy.* Thorofare, NJ: Slack Inc., 1988.

Time Reference Inventory

Roos P, Albers R: Performance of alcoholics and normals on a measure of temporal orientation. *J Clin Psych* 21: 34-36, 1965.

Occupational Performance History Interview

Kielhofner G, Henry AD, Walens D: *A User's Guide to the Occupational Performance History Interview.* Rockville, MD: American Occupational Therapy Association, 1989.

Test Publisher
American Occupational Therapy Association
1383 Piccard Drive
PO Box 1725
Rockville, MD 20849-1725

◆ TREATMENT LEVEL TWO EVALUATIONS ◆

COGNITIVE

Problem-Solving Inventory

Heppner PP, Petersen CH: The development and implications of a personal problem-solving inventory. *J Counsel Psych* 29: 66-75, 1982.

Automatic Thoughts Questionnaire

Hollon SD, Kendall PC: Cognitive self-statements in depression: Development of an automatic thoughts questionnaire. *Cog Ther Res* 4: 383-395, 1980.

PSYCHOLOGICAL

Hassles and Uplifts Scales

Lazarus R, Folkman S

Test Publisher
Consulting Psychologists Press, Inc.
577 College Ave.
Palo Alto, CA 94306

Ways of Coping Questionnaire

Lazarus R, Folkman S: *Stress, Appraisal, and Coping.* New York: Springer Publishing Co, 1984.

Test Publisher
Consulting Psychologists Press, Inc.
577 College Ave.
Palo Alto, CA 94306

COPE Inventory

Carver CS, Scheier MF, Weintraub JK: Assessing coping strategies: A theoretically based approach. *J Pers Soc Psychol* 56(2): 267-283, 1989.

Internal/External Scale

Rotter JB: Generalized expectancies for internal versus external control of reinforcement. *Psych Mon* 80: 1-28, 1966.

Coping Resources Inventory

Hammer AL, Marting MS: *Manual for the Coping Resources Inventory.* Palo Alto, CA: Consulting Psychologist Press, 1988.

Test Publisher
Consulting Psychologists Press, Inc.
577 College Ave.
Palo Alto, CA 94306

Coping Operations Preference Enquiry (COPE)

Schutz W

Test Publisher
Consulting Psychologists Press, Inc.
577 College Ave.
Palo Alto, CA 94306

Occupational Questionnaire

Smith NR, Kielhofner G, Watts JH: The relationships between volition, activity pattern and life satisfaction in the elderly. *AJOT* 40(4): 278-283, 1986.

SOCIAL

Social Reticence Scale

Jones WH, Russell D: The social reticence scale: An objective instrument to measure shyness. *J Pers Assess* 46: 629-631, 1982.

Test Publisher
Consulting Psychologists Press, Inc.
577 College Ave.
Palo Alto, CA 94306

Gambrill-Richey Assertion Inventory

Gambrill ED, Richey C: An assertion inventory for use in assessment and research. *Behav Ther* 6: 550-561, 1975.

Interpersonal Behavior Survey (IBS)

Mauger PA, Adkins DR, Zoss S, Frestone G, Hook D

Test Publisher
Western Psychological Service
12031 Wilshire Boulevard
Los Angeles, CA 90025

Social Skills Inventory

Riggio, RE

Test Publisher
Consulting Psychologists Press, Inc.
577 College Ave.
Palo Alto, CA 94306

Interpersonal Style Inventory (ISI)

Lorr M, Youniss R: An inventory of interpersonal style. *Tests of Personal Assessment* 37: 165-173, 1973.

Test Publisher
Western Psychological Service
12031 Wilshire Boulevard
Los Angeles, CA 90025

Social Climate Scales
 Moos RH: *Evaluating Treatment Environments: A Social Ecological Approach.* New York: Wiley, 1974.

 Moos RH: *Evaluating educational environments.* San Francisco: Jossey-Bass, 1979.

 Test Publisher
  Consulting Psychologists Press, Inc.
  577 College Ave.
  Palo Alto, CA 94306

The Role Checklist
 Oakley F, Kielhofner G, Barris R, Reichler RK: The role checklist: Development and empirical assessment of reliability. *Occ Ther J Res* 6(3): 157-169, 1986.

The Salience Inventory
 Super DE, Nevill DD

 Test Publisher
  Consulting Psychologists Press, Inc.
  577 College Ave.
  Palo Alto, CA 94306

Assessment of Occupational Functioning (AOF)
 Watts JH, Kielhofner G, Bauer DF, Gregory MD, Valentine DB: The assessment of occupational functioning: A screening tool for use in long-term care. *AJOT* 40(4): 231-240, 1986.

Occupational History
 Moorhead L: The occupational history. *AJOT* 23(4): 329-334, 1969.

Adolescent Role Assessment
 Black MM: Adolescent role assessment. *AJOT* 30: 73-79, 1982.

Role Activity Performance Scale
 Good-Ellis M, Fine SB, Spencer JH: Developing a role activity performance scale. *AJOT* 41(4): 232, 1985.

WORK

Independent Living Behavior Checklist
 Walls RT, Zane T, Thued JE: *Independent Living Behavior Checklist.* Morgantown, WV: West Virginia Rehabilitation Research and Training Center, 1979.

Kohlman Evaluation of Living Skills (KELS)
 Thomson, LK: *Kohlman evaluation of daily living skills (KELS).* Rockland, MD: AOTA, 1992.

 Test Publisher
  American Occupational Therapy Association
  1383 Piccard Drive
  PO Box 1725
  Rockville, MD 20849-1725

The Scorable Self-Care Evaluation (SSCE)

Peters M, Clark N: *Scorable Self-care Evaluation.* Thorofare, NJ: Slack Inc., 1984.

Test Publisher
Slack Inc.
6900 Grove Road
Thorofare, NJ 08086

The Work Behavior Checklist and the Occupational Therapy Vocational Skills Evaluation

Jacobs K: *Occupational Therapy: Work-related Programs and Assessments.* Boston, MA: Little, Brown and Company, 1985.

Rahim Organizational Conflict Inventories

Rahim MA: Measurement of organizational conflict. *J Gen Psych* 109: 189-199, 1983.

Test Publisher
Consulting Psychologists Press, Inc.
577 College Ave.
Palo Alto, CA 94306

LEISURE

Kohlman Evaluation of Living Skills (KELS)

Thomson, LK: *Kohlman evaluation of daily living skills (KELS).* Rockland, MD: AOTA, 1992.

Test Publisher
American Occupational Therapy Association
1383 Piccard Drive
PO Box 1725
Rockville, MD 20849-1725

The Scorable Self-Care Evaluation (SSCE)

Peters M, Clark N: *Scorable Self-care Evaluation.* Thorofare, NJ: Slack Inc., 1984

Test Publisher
Slack Inc.
6900 Grove Road
Thorofare, NJ 08086

Interest Checklist

Matsutsuyu J: The interest checklist. *AJOT* 11: 179-181, 1967.

Rogers J, Weinstein J, Firone J: The interest checklist: An empirical assessment. *AJOT* 32: 628-630, 1978.

Leisure Activities Blank

Morgan A, Bodbey G: The effect of entering an age-segregated environment upon the leisure activity pattern of older adults. *J Leis Res* 10: 77-190, 1978.

Leisure Satisfaction Scale

Beard J, Ragheb M: Measuring leisure satisfaction. *J Leis Res* 12: 20-33, 1980.

HOMEMAKING/PARENTING

Comprehensive Evaluation of Basic Living Skills (CEBLS)

Casanova JS, Ferber J: Comprehensive evaluation of basic living skills. *AJOT* 30: 101-105, 1976.

Kohlman Evaluation of Living Skills (KELS)

Thomson, LK: *Kohlman evaluation of daily living skills (KELS)*. Rockland, MD: AOTA, 1992.

Test Publisher
American Occupational Therapy Association
1383 Piccard Drive
PO Box 1725
Rockville, MD 20849-1725

The Scorable Self-Care Evaluation (SSCE)

Peters M, Clark N: *Scorable Self-care Evaluation*. Thorofare, NJ: Slack Inc., 1984

Test Publisher
Slack Inc.
6900 Grove Road
Thorofare, NJ 08086

Independent Living Skills Evaluation

Johnson TP, Vinnicombe BJ, Merril GW: The independent living skills evaluation. *Occup Ther Men Hea* 1(2): 5-18, 1980.

Independent Living Behavior Checklist

Walls RT, Zane T, Thued JE: *Independent Living Behavior Checklist*. Morgantown, WV: West Virginia Rehabilitation Research and Training Center, 1979.

RELAPSE

Coping Resources Inventory

Hammer AL, Marting MS: *Manual for the Coping Resources Inventory*. Palo Alto, CA: Consulting Psychologist Press, 1988.

Test Publisher
Consulting Psychologists Press, Inc.
577 College Ave.
Palo Alto, CA 94306

Problem Situation Inventory

Hawkins JD, Catalano RF, Wells EA: Measuring effects of a skills training intervention for drug abusers. *J Consul Clin Psych* 54(5): 661-664, 1986.

Hawkins JD, Catalano RF, Gillmore MR, Wells EA: Skills training for drug abusers: Generalization, maintenance, and effects on drug use. *J Consul Clin Psych* 57(4): 559-563, 1989.

Environmental Questionnaire

Dunning HD: Environmental occupational therapy. *AJOT* 26: 292-298, 1972.

Pleasant Events Schedule

MacPhillamy JD, Lewinsohn PM: *Manual for the Pleasant Events Schedule*. Eugene, OR: Department of Psychology, University of Oregon.

MacPhillamy JD, Lewinsohn PM: The pleasant events schedule: Studies on reliability, validity, and scale intercorrelations. *J Consul Clin Psych* 50: 363-380, 1982.

◆ TREATMENT LEVEL THREE EVALUATIONS ◆

PSYCHOLOGICAL

Azima Battery

Hemphill B (Ed): *The Evaluative Process in Psychiatric Occupational Therapy*. Thorofare, NJ: Slack Inc., 1982.

BH Battery

Hemphill B: *Training Manual for the BH Battery*. Thorofare NJ: Slack Inc., 1982.

Test Publisher
Slack Inc.
6900 Grove Road
Thorofare, NJ 08086

Fidler Battery

Fidler G, Fidler J: *Occupational Therapy: A Communicative Process in Psychiatry*. New York: The Macmillan CO, 1963.

Goodman Battery

Hemphill B (Ed): *The Evaluative Process in Psychiatric Occupational Therapy*. Thorofare, NJ: Slack Inc., 1982.

Magazine Picture Collage

Lerner CJ: The magazine picture collage: Its clinical use and validity as an assessment device. *Am J Occup Ther* 33: 500-504, 1979.

Lerner CJ, Ross G: The magazine picture collage: Development of an objective scoring system. *Am J Occup Ther* 31: 156-161, 1977.

Buck R, Provancher M: Magazine picture collage as an evaluation technique. *Am J Occup Ther* 26: 36-39, 1972.

Shoemyen Battery

Shoemyen C: Occupational therapy orientation and media. *Am J Occup Ther* 24: 276-279, 1970.

Hemphill B (Ed): *The Evaluative Process in Psychiatric Occupational Therapy*. Thorofare, NJ: Slack Inc., 1982.

Coopersmith Self-Esteem Inventories

Coopersmith S: *Self-esteem Inventories*. Palo Alto, CA: 1981.

Test Publisher
Consulting Psychologists Press, Inc.
577 College Ave.
Palo Alto, CA 94306

Tennessee Self-Concept Scale

Fitts WH: *Manual: Tennessee Self-Concept Scale*. Los Angeles: Western Psychological Services, 1965.

Test Publisher
Western Psychological Service
12031 Wilshire Boulevard
Los Angeles, CA 90025

Self-Esteem Scale

Rosenberg M: *Society and the Adolescent Self-image*. Princeton, NJ: Princeton University Press, 1965.

Robinson J, Shaver P: *Measures of Social Psychological Attitudes*. Ann Arbor, MI: Institute of Social Research, 1973, pp. 81-83.

VALUES

Projective Techniques

Hemphill B (Ed): *The Evaluative Process in Psychiatric Occupational Therapy*. Thorofare, NJ: Slack Inc., 1982.

Mosey AC: *Psychosocial Components of Occupational Therapy*. New York: Raven Press, 1986.

Life Purpose Questionnaire (LPQ)

Hutzell RR, Peterson TJ: Use of the life purpose questionnaire with an alcoholic population. *Int J Addict* 21(1): 51-57, 1986.

Occupational Case Analysis Interview and Rating Scale (OCAIRS)

Kaplan KL, Kielhofner G: *Occupational Case Analysis Interview and Rating Scale*. Thorofare, NJ: Slack Inc., 1989.

Test Publisher
Slack Inc.
6900 Grove Road
Thorofare, NJ 08086

Occupational Role History

Florey L, Michelman SM: The occupational role history: A screening tool for psychiatric occupational therapy. *AJOT* 36(5): 301-308.

The Role Checklist

Oakley F, Kielhofner G, Barris R, Reichler RK: The role checklist: Development and empirical assessment of reliability. *Occ Ther J Res* 6(3): 157-169, 1986.

The Salience Inventory

Super DE, Nevill DD

Test Publisher
Consulting Psychologists Press, Inc.
577 College Ave.
Palo Alto, CA 94306

The Rokeach Value Survey

Rokeach M: *Values Survey*. Sunnyvale, CA: Halgren Tests, 1967.

Test Publisher
Consulting Psychologists Press, Inc.
577 College Ave.
Palo Alto, CA 94306

California Life Goals Evaluation Schedules

Hahn ME: *California Life Goals Evaluation Schedules Manual*. Los Angeles: Western Psychological Service, 1969.

Test Publisher
Western Psychological Service
12031 Wilshire Boulevard
Los Angeles, CA 90025

Personal Orientation Inventory

Shostrom EL: *Personal Orientation Inventory (POI) Manual*. San Diego, CA: EDITS, 1966 & 1974.

EXPANDED ROLES

Michill Adjective Rating Scale (MARS)

Quereshi MY: The development of the Michill Adjective Rating Scale (MARS). *J Clin Psychol* 26: 192-196, 1970.

Adolescent Role Assessment

Black MM: Adolescent role assessment. *AJOT* 30: 73-79, 1982.

Occupational Role History

Florey L, Michelman SM: The occupational role history: A screening tool for psychiatric occupational therapy. *AJOT* 36(5): 301-308.

The Role Checklist

Oakley F, Kielhofner G, Barris R, Reichler RK: The role checklist: Development and empirical assessment of reliability. *Occ Ther J Res* 6(3): 157-169, 1986.

The Salience Inventory
Super DE, Nevill DD

Test Publisher
Consulting Psychologists Press, Inc.
577 College Ave.
Palo Alto, CA 94306

Index